Harper's BAZAAR

Great Style

Great

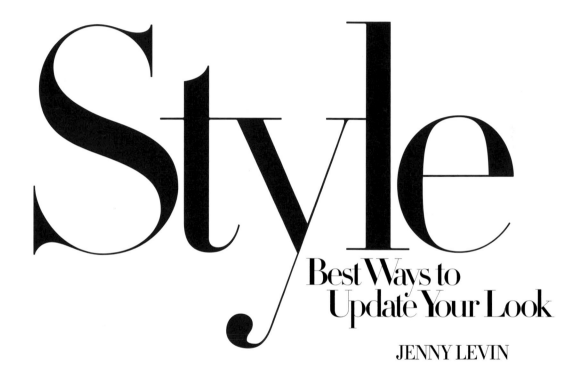

Style

Best Ways to Update Your Look

JENNY LEVIN

HEARST BOOKS
A division of Sterling Publishing Co., Inc.

New York / London
www.sterlingpublishing.com

Contents

Foreword 6

1 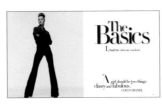 The Basics 8

2 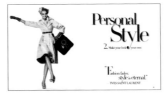 Personal Style 28

3 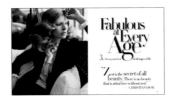 Fabulous at Every Age 50

4 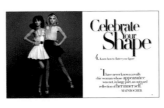 Celebrate Your Shape 78

5 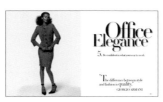 Office Elegance 100

6 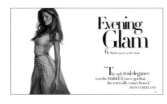 Evening Glam 124

7 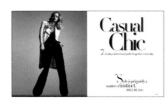 Casual Chic 154

8 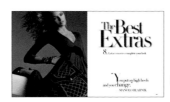 The Best Extras 192

9 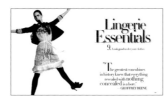 Lingerie Essentials 220

The Last Word 232
Index 234
Photo Credits 238

Foreword

I love giving fashion advice. Not only is it my job—and I love my job—it's also my personal mission to give fashion advice to anyone who wants a little help. After all, if we have nothing to fear but fear itself, then the only way to be a fashion victim is to fear fashion.

This year, to mark our 140th anniversary, *Bazaar* has put together this book, featuring the best of what we do best: sharing the secrets to looking great, from dressing appropriately for your age and shape to shopping like an expert.

At *Bazaar*, we firmly believe fashion should be fun. Can you think of anything else that instantly makes you look and feel like a million and brings you so much joy (without a prescription)? But what works at 25 can look not so hot after 40. Luckily, there are hundreds of ways to be fabulous at every age, and we've got them all right here for you.

Being chic is about dressing appropriately for all occasions but also about standing out from the pack. The legendary

Coco Chanel once said, "Look for the woman in the dress. If there is no woman, there is no dress." Wearing the same designer from head to toe says everything about the designer and nothing about you, so we've asked some of the world's best-dressed women to offer their tips on how to look effortlessly chic.

Whether you want to learn to build the perfect wardrobe, what to wear when, ways to dress to flatter your figure, or when to splurge and when to save, these pages are packed with practical advice for making your personal style work for your lifestyle.

Legendary *Bazaar* editor Diana Vreeland once declared, "You gotta have style. It helps you get up in the morning. It's a way of life."

As America's first fashion magazine, *Bazaar* has always been for the well-dressed woman with a well-dressed mind, and this book has been designed to help you be just that.

Enjoy.

Glenda

Glenda Bailey
Editor in Chief
Harper's Bazaar

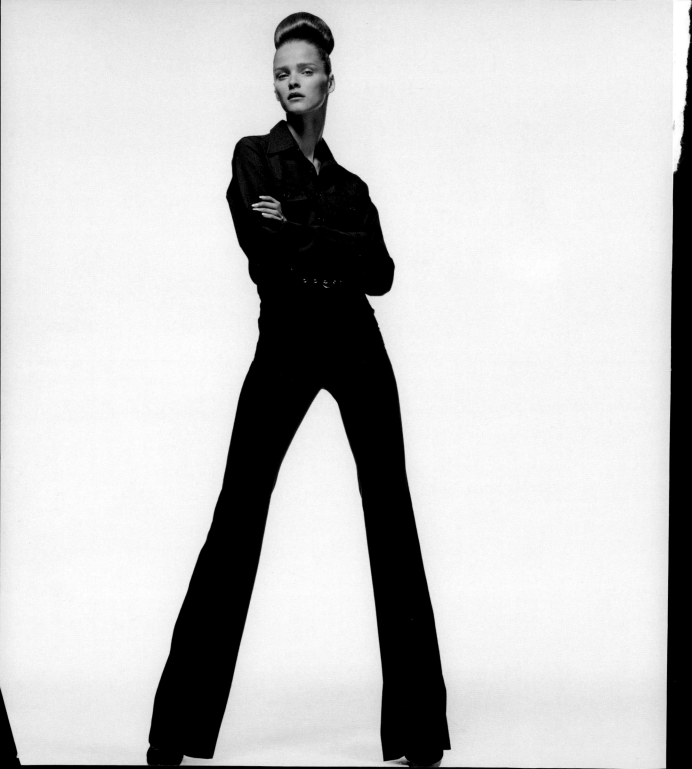

The Basics

1. Build the ultimate wardrobe

"A girl should be two things: classy and fabulous."

—COCO CHANEL

Every day, sometimes two or three times, you open those closet doors and think, What am I going to wear? Occasionally, due to the excitement over a recent purchase or a specific event, the answer is an easy one: "Ooh … I'm going to debut my new dress" or "I have a meeting with the boss and *must* have on my lucky power suit." But most of the time, it's the age-old lament: "I have nothing to wear." So you end up standing in front of the closet for what seems like eons trying to figure out what will be perfect for that day, considering your current mood, the weather, and the moment. Worse yet, you go through multiple try-ons and inevitably end up running late for work, unsatisfied and with a pile of clothes on the bed to come home to. But all is not lost. There is a way out of this clothes quagmire, and a properly stocked closet, filled with all the right basics, is the place to start.

Closet Essentials

The five pieces every woman should own

No wardrobe is complete without certain tried-and-true staples that work as the foundations for any look. Here, the fashion necessities for the well-rounded, well-dressed woman. Use these key items as your building blocks:

1. A dark—preferably black—lean suit

The jacket and trousers can be worn separately for more mileage.

2. A pencil skirt

This can be A-line if it's more flattering for your body type but should be simple and refined.

3. A crisp white shirt

Dressed up or down, it will always be chic.

4. A great pair of jeans

A straight cut in a darker wash is more versatile.

5. A little black dress

Also called the LBD, it will never let you down.

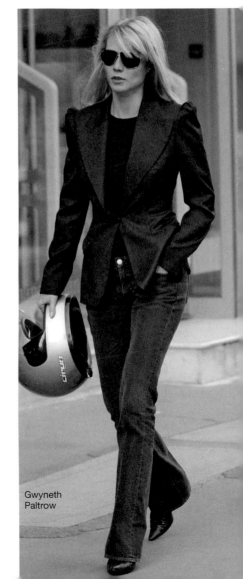

Gwyneth
Paltrow

Ultimate Classics

The timeless staples

Once you have your closet essentials down, it's worth stocking up on pieces that will always look great, no matter the trend du jour. Think versatility, longevity, and everlasting appeal—the clothing that style setters from Catherine Deneuve to Kate Moss have always relied on.

- **White tees:** They are the all-American standard. You'll always find uses for basic tees, whether atop denim on weekends or with a dressy skirt for a sporty edge. They're also the groundwork for layering.

- **Cashmere cardigans:** As part of a sweater set or in a longer V-neck grandpa cut, a button-up sweater offers the most adaptability—perfect with a pencil skirt for work, sexy at night with nothing underneath or as a cocktail-dress topper, and a great layering piece for casual days. Classic colors—camel, navy, black, and gray—will inevitably get more wear than brights or patterns.

- **White jeans:** A more glamorous take on basic jeans, these clean pants are effortless cool epitomized. All they need is a cashmere V-neck on top for a jet-set aura. They even work in the winter paired with a cozy knit or fur. (Very après ski!)

- **Trousers:** Channel Katharine Hepburn with classic slouchy pants. They're all about refined ease. Wear them with a soft blouse, a crisp button-up, or a thin knit.

- **Shift dress:** Think Jackie O's simple, pared-down, but polished style. The minimal frock couldn't be easier to wear—working with a blouse or a tee under, with flats or pumps—making it a no-brainer for every woman's wardrobe.

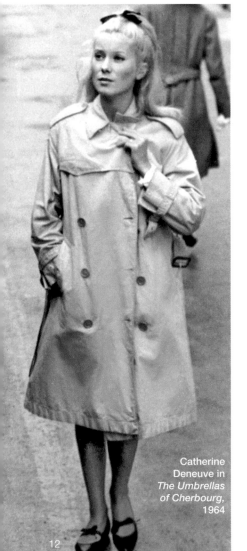

Catherine Deneuve in *The Umbrellas of Cherbourg,* 1964

- # Tuxedo: Just as the LBD will always work for evening affairs, the tuxedo, or *le smoking,* is a dashing alternative. With the allure of being covered up and the whole masculine-feminine mix, a tux at night can be utterly sexy. Bonus: A slim suit can be extremely flattering for all body types.

- # Bouclé jacket: Coco Chanel made this a wardrobe must. Worn with a matching skirt or with jeans, the tweedy jacket, boxy or fitted, adds instant luxe.

- # Trench coat: It's the ultimate symbol of chic— loved by women young, old, curvy, slim, conservative, or edgy. It's a versatile piece that is at the same time practical, glamorous, and cool. Whether you wear it over worn-in jeans or a fancy dress, you're sure to look sophisticated.

- # Camel overcoat: A coat is the first and last thing people see on you, so it's worth finding a plush one, but keeping it sleek and classic increases its life span and wearability. You can't go wrong with a cashmere coat in deep tan, whether it's a wrap version or double- or single-breasted. It works day and night, for work and weekends.

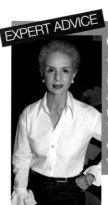
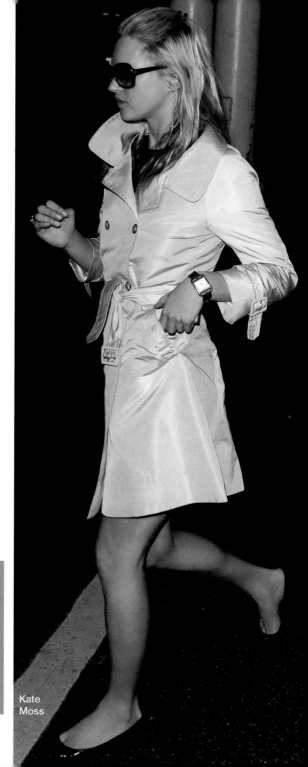

Kate Moss

Enduring Chic

A look at iconic pieces that have stood the test of time

There are some items of clothing that are impervious to trends and never fail to look good, no matter what year it is. Wearing one of these ever-stylish standards, you're sure to feel confidently well dressed, always.

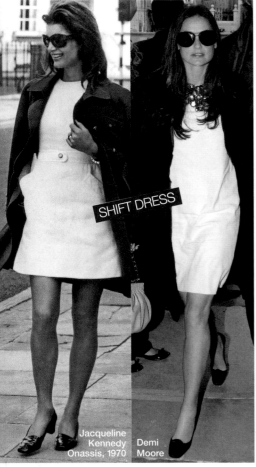

SHIFT DRESS

Jacqueline Kennedy Onassis, 1970

Demi Moore

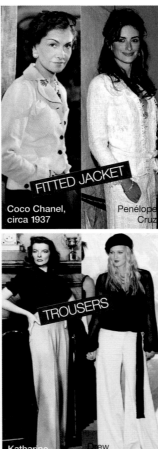

FITTED JACKET

Coco Chanel, circa 1937

Penélope Cruz

TROUSERS

Katharine Hepburn, 1940

Drew Barrymore

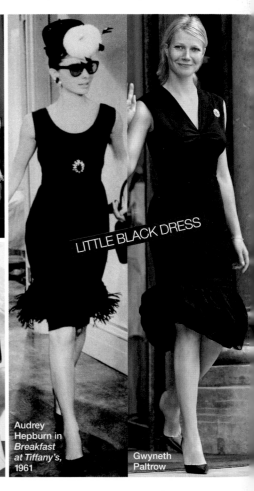

LITTLE BLACK DRESS

Audrey Hepburn in *Breakfast at Tiffany's*, 1961

Gwyneth Paltrow

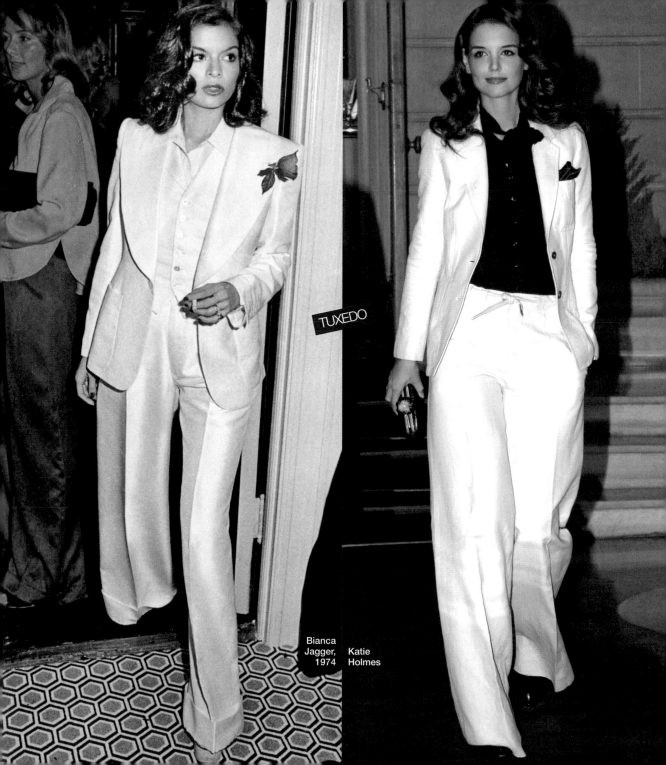

TUXEDO

Bianca
Jagger,
1974

Katie
Holmes

The Best Investment Pieces

What's worth spending on

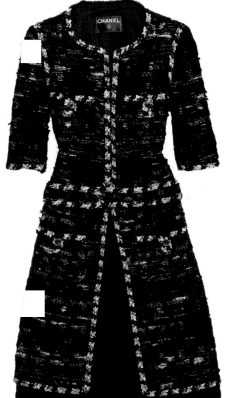

While it's never easy to spend big money on clothes, there are some things for which it makes sense to pay a little more. The key is to find high-quality, überversatile items like coats, cocktail dresses, and furs that defy fashion's mercurial moods. You'll end up getting so much wear out of these elite pieces that it's worth the price in the end. Think of it this way: Let's say you pay $1,000 for a cashmere coat. Since it's well made, you are likely to have it for a lifetime (okay, at least five years) and wear it about 150 days of the year (mostly in the fall and winter). That equals less than $1.50 per wear! Apply this fashion math to any of your big-ticket purchases. Here's where it makes sense to splurge.

- **Coat:** A streamlined cut that works over both casual and evening ensembles is worth the money. Look for superior fabric that will hold up to the elements. You want your coat to be a workhorse, but it should always look pristine.

- **Chunky knits:** High-quality cashmere looks better, lasts longer, and feels cozier. In the right shapes—cardigans, crewnecks, turtlenecks, and V-necks—sumptuous sweaters can luxe up any pair of jeans or cords and give a pair of trousers a softer, more laid-back feel.

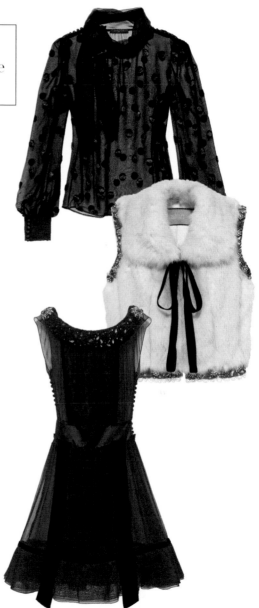

- **Blouses:** They're on top, so everyone notices them. Cheap fabrics look tacky and, well, cheap. Choose frills, ruffles, florals, or something sculpted, but whatever style you pick, it's best to go high-end with this prominent piece.

- **Fur:** Whether real or faux, a mink, sable, or fox (to name a few) jacket, coat, vest, or even scarf is the ultimate in luxury. Indulging in something top-of-the-line is the only way to get a lifetime of wear and then some. (Your children will thank you.) A shorter cut is recommended over full-length so you'll get better use out of it. (Wear it day and night.)

- **Cocktail dress:** You want to love your dress because you'll be relying on it quite often, and you'll want to feel confident and fabulous every time you put it on. It should fit you to perfection and have an air of elegance with a hint of sexiness.

- **Evening gown:** Perhaps you'll go formal once a year, but when you do, you want to radiate, be a knockout, be a princess for a night—and a short frock just won't fly. Whether you want something slinky, beaded, or grand, the material, makeup, and fit should be your highest priorities.

Great Finds

The pieces you can save on

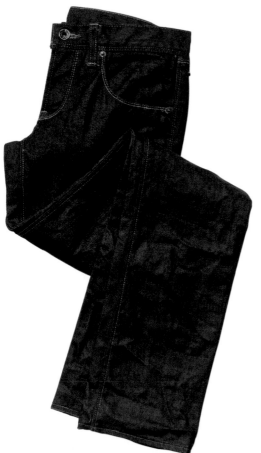

Luckily, when you're wardrobe building, there are many places where you can skimp a tad. It's not about low quality, it's about knowing what should be easy on the budget.

• **Jeans:** While, hands down, most people claim to get more wear out of their jeans than any other article of clothing, there is still no need to spend big bucks on your blues. Yes, we all have our favorites that get a lot of use, but we are also fickle and no doubt happier to have more than one cut to choose from—at least a pair to wear with high heels and one to wear with flats. Besides, who needs high-maintenance denim? You won't think twice about throwing more affordable jeans in the washer and dryer.

• **Pants:** Think of them in terms of dinner-table dressing. No one sees your bottom when you're sitting at a table, behind a desk, or even having a tête-à-tête at a crowded party. So why empty out your wallet on something that gets so little attention? Spend on your top. If that's exquisite, it'll keep all eyes up.

• **Skirts:** Following the same logic as pants, skirts are the second half of your outfit and are a support for your top, therefore they don't always have to be so pricey. Yet, unlike pants, they have the potential to define you— say, tantalizing in a thigh-high, demure in a dirndl, or powerful in a pencil—so choose your skirt shape wisely.

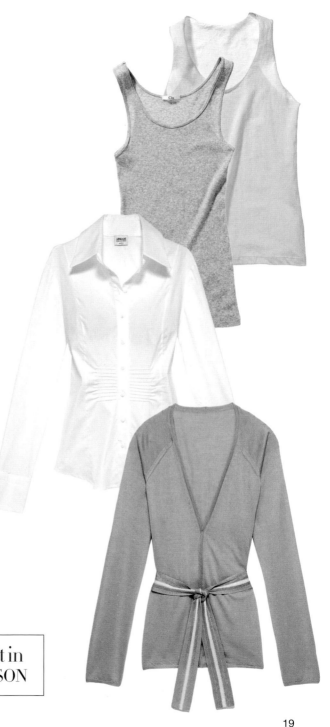

- **Button-ups:** These no-frills tops aren't meant to last a lifetime. White is the color of choice for the men's-style shirt, which means it needs to be laundered a lot. And it requires ironing to keep it neat. Therefore, the shirt gets worn out fast. Since it is best sharp and crisp, you'll want to restock often.

- **Lightweight knits:** Thin sweaters are ideal for layering, so it's advisable to have many in your stable. Because you'll use these as flexible go-to items (over anything, under some things, thrown in your bag in case you get cold), multi-ply, heavy-duty fabrics are not necessary. Fine (and therefore less expensive) wool or cotton works best.

- **Tees & tanks:** This is the most obvious area where you can pinch pennies. There are plenty of brands out there offering well-made tees with appropriate price tags. Look for longer styles for more layering versatility. So, when you find the best fit and fabric, stock up!

> "If you find something you like, get it in two colors." —ELLE MACPHERSON

How Many...

What should you *really* have in your wardrobe?

Here's a breakdown of the fundamentals of a well-stocked closet.
(Note: This is the bare minimum. Of course, there is nothing wrong with having more!)

4 sweaters
(2 workworthy and 2 for weekends)

7 tees
(short and long sleeves, tanks, and turtlenecks)

4 coats and jackets
(1 elegant coat, 1 sporty outerwear jacket, 1 classic trench, and 1 day-to-night jacket)

2 tops for every skirt and pant
(1 dressed-up and 1 casual style)

4 pants, 4 skirts
(2 office and evening appropriate and 2 informal)

1 suit
(for every season, that you can wear together or apart)

5 dresses
(2 for day, 1 short for cocktails, 1 long for formal, and 1 special knock-'em-dead frock)

4 jeans
(1 slim cut for a cleaner look, 1 relaxed fit for laid-back days, 1 ankle length for flats, and 1 longer pair for higher heels)

Make the Most of Your Wardrobe

How to get your clothes to go the distance

These days, it's a lucky few who have the funds to purchase a whole new wardrobe each season. Most of us, however, are a bit more limited and usually want to take full advantage of the clothes we buy—and wear them all year round. The trick is to make most of your clothes seasonless.

Suit up. The traditional two-piece can be a multipurpose wonder. Worn as a set, it's a work staple, but it also can be a sexy evening number when worn with a slinky camisole (or nothing) underneath. The skirt or pants can go on their own for any occasion— dressed up or dressed down. And the jacket is guaranteed to be sharp atop jeans or even a cocktail dress or gown.

Get creative. Experiment with letting your clothes live outside their designated roles. A classic white shirt, for example, while always great under a jacket, is also incredibly glam paired with a ball gown, tucked into jeans, and as a bathing-suit cover-up. Your trench can make a sexy nighttime option in a pinch when accessorized right. (Strappy heels are just about all you need.) Don't be afraid to turn your basics into something bold.

Arm yourself with tees. A long-sleeved tee or turtleneck can turn a warm-weather top or sundress into a sweet fall or winter look. Play with different weights and fabrics. Even a simple cotton tank can give a new mood to a dress. Have a white dress you want to wear when the mercury drops? Throw a black turtleneck underneath. In addition, layering under a dress can make something slinky okay to wear during the day. Tees and tanks also come in handy to lighten up a heavy trouser or skirt.

Embrace knits. Clearly, cardigans (chunky or lightweight) can give any summery outfit a cozier feel. And they'll never fail for cooler evenings. But knits can also work as underpinnings. Try a woolly piece under a shift for a '70s Ali MacGraw–worthy air.

> "I've always admired a woman who can dress for all occasions—someone who's not fashion crazy, but you always want to look like her." —RALPH LAUREN

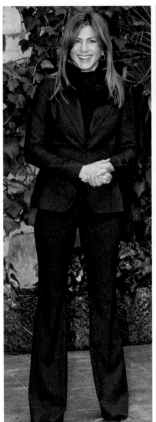
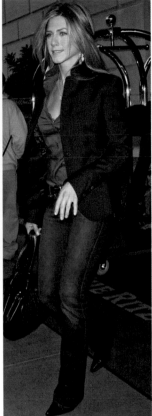
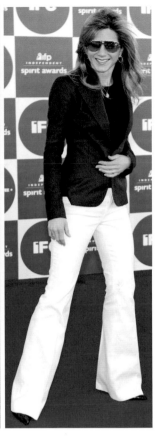

3 Ways to Wear a Blazer

Classic dresser Jennifer Aniston knows the value of a good suit. The traditional twosome looks smart as a set, but the jacket alone is just as chic.

A dark suit: You can rest assured you'll look appropriate—say, at work or on evenings out—in a sleek suit. Try a classic, frill-free cut and avoid getting caught up in short-lived trends. Plus, black will always be flattering. Find a cut that works for you and stick with it.

A jacket & jeans: Your favorite blues with a tailored jacket is what casual chic is all about. A fitted jacket (Aniston seems to favor the one-button cut) is the most polished.

A mismatched suit: Try your suit blazer with different trousers. A wide-leg style in crisp white, for example, is dressier than denim and a nice alternative in warmer weather.

January

- Scour *Harper's Bazaar* for a preview of the best looks from designers' spring lines.
- Secure your spot on the waitlists for the most covetable pieces.
- Couture collections are shown in Paris. Look for trends that you can work into your own wardrobe.

February

- Spring clothes land in stores. Look out for the season's key pieces.
- Assess your wardrobe and determine what pieces are missing or need refreshing.
- Act fast: The best shoes and bags sell out first.
- Fall fashions debut in New York, Milan, and Paris.

March

- Spring fashion is in high gear in stores and in the magazines.
- Tear pages from magazines of your favorite pieces to help you shop.
- Check the Internet for the fall collections. Pick your favorite looks now.

A Shopping Calendar:

July

- Get your first peek at the newest trends and essential pieces for fall in *Bazaar*.
- Call stores and secure your favorite pieces now, before they hit the shelves.
- It's Paris couture time again. Look on the Internet to see what develops.

August

- Fall fashions hit stores. Pull out the to-buy list you made in February and run to your favorite shops.
- Check your closet to see what cold-weather items need new life. Do your boots need resoling? Time to buy a new coat?

September

- The new season is at its peak. Fill in your wardrobe with fall's best suits, jackets, and coats.
- Don't forget to score the It bag, shoe, and boots!
- Spring collections make their runway debut in New York, Milan, and Paris.

What to Buy When

April

- Time to transition into your lightweight wardrobe.
- Try swapping your suits for springy dresses.
- Buy a trench! If you have a classic khaki already, get a new one in black or crisp white.

May

- Start thinking summer! Pull out your sandals, shorts, and sundresses from storage and see what needs to be updated or refurbished.
- Don't put it off: Get out there and shop for a new swimsuit. Give yourself time to find the perfect one.

June

- Prefall lines are in stores. It's a good time to buy basics and classics.
- Stay chic in the heat with breezy pieces and strategic layering.
- Summer-sales alert! Scour the racks for any designer goodies you may have missed out on.

October

- Spruce up your wardrobe with extra touches, whether that means cool jewelry, fun belts, or sexy shoes.
- Buy your LBD and all your evening accoutrements now. The holidays will be here sooner than you think.
- Sales alert: Look out for deals on coats and cashmere.

November

- While you should start making headway on your gift lists, think about personal pieces like lingerie. You know you could use some new unmentionables.
- Make sure you have everything in order for all the parties next month.

December

- It's all about the holidays, and shopping is at a fever pitch. Don't forget to buy something for yourself.
- Resort collections make a splash in stores. Now's the perfect time to buy for warm-weather vacations.

Shop Like an Expert

Scouring the racks? Hauling bags around? Waiting in line at the registers? Who has time? Shopping should be sweet and simple. The answer? Consider yourself a VIP and take advantage of the tricks celebrities utilize. Personal service is there for the taking— and guess what? It's free.

When it comes to stocking up on all your major purchases, forget trolling racks to find your size, running from floor to floor to put a look together, waving down an inattentive salesperson, or lugging bags around all day. Just have someone do it for you. Don't worry, you don't need a celebrity paycheck; most major shops and department stores offer personal shopping at no extra cost. The process couldn't be easier. A private session usually starts with a conversation about your likes, sizes, needs, and budget, followed by an appointment lasting anywhere from one to four hours. And when you arrive at the store, voilà, you'll have a stocked dressing room waiting and you're ready to start wardrobe building. Your fashion pro will ensure everything fits (and is tailored right there) and offer advice on mixing and matching, accessorizing, and what to wear when. Not only are instant alterations key to efficient shopping, having your bags shipped or delivered home when you've still got a lot of shopping to do is worth the typically nominal fees.

While being pampered is certainly something we all could use, many of us just want to get our shopping done as fast as possible. In the busy lives of women today, saving time is the real treat. Well, perhaps the ultimate luxury in shopping would be not shopping at all, but learning to shop deftly and efficiently will make the difference between a failed closet-restocking mission and a successful one.

Time-Saving Shopping Tips

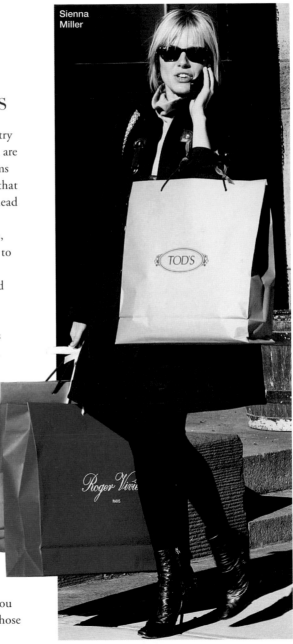

Sienna Miller

- **Set up an appointment** with a personal shopper and try to be as specific as possible about what you expect and are looking for. Bring clips from fashion magazines of items you like or actual pieces you are looking to refresh. If that sounds too high maintenance for you, try calling ahead so a staffer can prepare a dressing room for you.
- **Go solo.** Husbands, boyfriends, girlfriends, mothers, and children can be distractions when getting down to the business of wardrobe building.
- **Have your clothes altered** at the time of purchase and sent to your house or office.
- **Build a relationship with an insider** at your favorite store. He or she will pull pieces for you, hold hot items for you or put your name on the waitlist for them, and call you when popular pieces come in. Touch base with your in-store friend regularly.
- **Keep your credit card on file** at trusted stores so you can avoid the wait at the register. (Some small boutiques will even offer house accounts to their big-spending and loyal customers.) That way you can get your shopping done in a flash—or even make purchases over the phone.
- **Shop at off-peak hours.** When the store first opens is best; everything is neat and orderly, and you'll have a salesperson all to yourself. Avoid the lunchtime and postwork rushes.
- **Take care of those who take care of you.** Thank-you notes, holiday gifts, and a general appreciation for those who've helped you will go a long way.

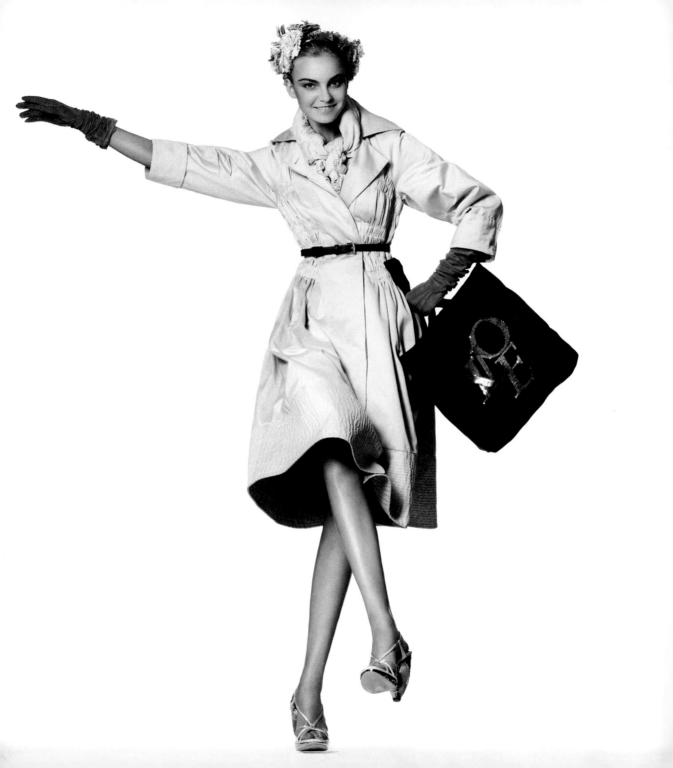

Personal Style

2. Make your look your own

"Fashion fades; style is eternal."
—YVES SAINT LAURENT

Some say there is an art to dressing well. That may be true. Mastering what goes with what, knowing which designers are in and which are out, and eyeing exactly where the hemline should hit and how high the heel should be certainly take talent. But let's face it, most us don't have the time, energy, or patience to elevate what we wear every day to an art form. Our goal is to feel comfortable, confident, and chic in the clothes we put on. We want dressing to be effortless—and we want to look effortlessly dressed. Yes, there are the enviable lucky few who have a knack for looking oh-so-perfectly pulled together every time they step out the door, and then there are the rest of us, who have to try a little harder (and still those who don't bother at all). But with the proper tools, the right mind-set, and a little direction from the fashion icons of the world, we all can be well dressed all the time.

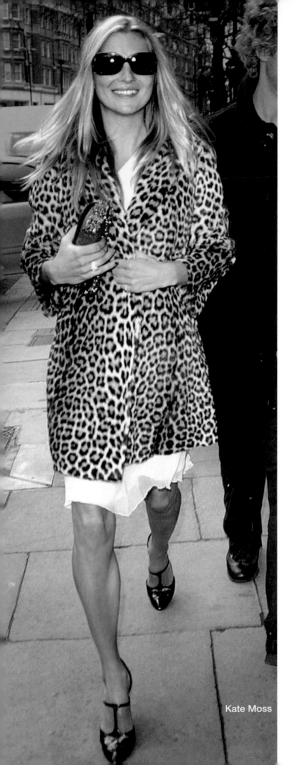
Kate Moss

Express Your Inner Fashion Sense

Learn to find the style star in you

The trick to looking fashionable is not simply wearing the best pieces from the runways—although it's a start. Real style is *how* you wear them, putting your own stamp on the outfit you choose to wear. It's the little twists on the trends, the nuances, and the added élan that make all the difference. You want to create an air of individuality and separate yourself from the fashion pack. Personal style should be your goal when it comes to dressing.

Here, tips to finding your own style:

- **Don't dress in a look** straight off the runway or all in one trend.
- **Feel free to mix** and match.
- **Don't be stuck** on one style; experiment with new looks. Or, find a signature look and be true to it.
- **If you like it,** buy it and wear it—with confidence.
- **Have fun with trends,** but don't be a slave to them.
- **Know that keeping it simple** is often the best way to go.
- **Add your own touch** to a look, whether it's a bow, belt, or brooch.
- **Do the unexpected.** Don't always wear things in the traditional way.

"The advice I now give: Never wear a designer look head to toe. —KATE MOSS

Fashion
Personalities

Our clothes are often an expression of our spirit and character, so there is nothing wrong with finding a look that suits you and relying on it. What category best characterizes you?

The most stylish women in the world are surprisingly consistent in what they wear every day, whether that means keeping to basics or getting creative all the time. Some are known for a classic aesthetic, others bohemian. There are those who are not afraid to be edgy and those who prefer a more ladylike way of dressing. No matter which signature look best describes them, they've found something they feel confident in and stuck with it. These women seem to have dressing down pat and look comfortable and secure in their clothes—and that's what we all strive for. Here is a peek at fashion icons and the style that best sums them up. Where do you fit in?

Jacqueline Kennedy
Onassis, 1974

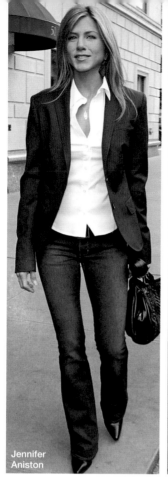

Jennifer
Aniston

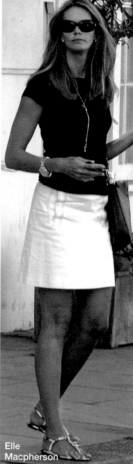

Elle
Macpherson

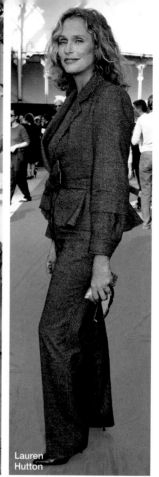

Lauren
Hutton

The Classicists

These women prefer basics—the T-shirt, blazer, white shirt, suit, and trousers—and look effortlessly chic in simple staple pieces

- **Embrace tradition.** Sticking with things that have stood the test of time is often the key to looking clean and elegant.
- **Say "no thanks" to trends.** The hottest and newest don't always suit a simpler style. If intrigued by a trend, incorporate it into your look in a subtle way, maybe with an accessory.

- **Keep a clean line.** Frivolity, frills, and fanciful cuts are not in tune with a more established approach to dressing.
- **Pick a pared-down palette.** Black, white, navy, gray, and khaki are classic. When going for color, stick to print-free pieces in straightforward shapes.

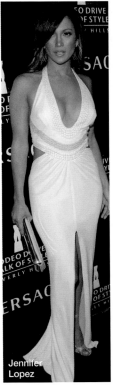

Jennifer Lopez

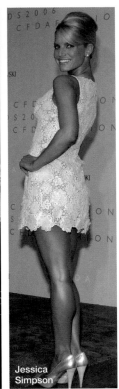

Jessica Simpson

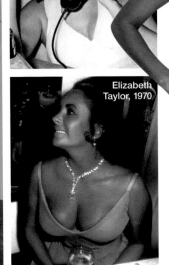

Sophia Loren, circa 1964

Elizabeth Taylor, 1970

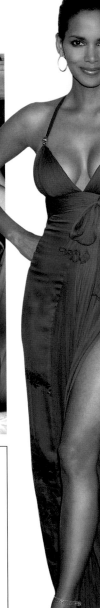

Halle Berry

The Bombshells

Sexy is the mantra for these women. And for them, picking pieces that show off a curvy, feminine figure is the norm.

- **Look for clothes that accentuate the hourglass.** Deep V's and high slits are de rigueur.
- **Choose body-hugging, figure-flattering cuts.** Avoid sack dresses, dirndls, masculine tailoring, and anything with too much coverage.

- **Brights, white, and black** all work in solid shades. Prints, patterns, and elaborate embellishment detract from the focal point, your body.
- **Wallflowers need not apply.** When dressing like a sultry siren, be prepared to draw attention to yourself.

The Bohemians

Bell-bottoms may have given way to breezy gowns, but these free-spirited style setters love earthy, ethnic-inspired looks

- **Stay chic.** Dressing like a modern-day flower child isn't license to look sloppy.
- **Master the mix.** Layering pieces, pairing new with vintage, and combining multiple textures all add to the appeal.
- **Banish plain shades.** Wearing a rainbow of colors highlights a carefree demeanor.
- **Play up prints.** Swirly paisleys, pretty florals, retro patterns—the haute-hippie chick can pull off funky patterns.

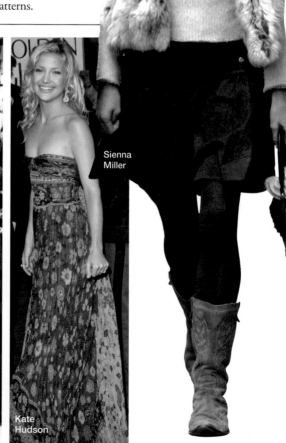

Sienna Miller

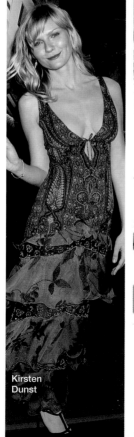

Kirsten Dunst

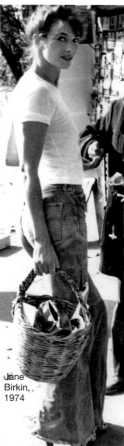

Jane Birkin, 1974

Kate Hudson

The Ladies

Grace Kelly's white-glove look may be a little old-fashioned, but her prim, polished, and pulled-together air still resonates with today's refined set

- **Keep it feminine but not flirty.** Pick a silhouette that shows off your waist but not too much else. If you want to show some skin, choose one erogenous zone—like your shoulders, ankles, or décolletage—at a time.
- **Add charm.** A bow, a touch of lace, or a slight ruffle offers a sweet edge. But keep it to one or two flourishes.

- **Classic colors are most appropriate.** Black and white will never fail you. Avoid anything over-the-top or garish. If you want to add color, try a red shoe or lip.
- **Fabric counts.** Look for structured, high-quality materials. Anything too flimsy or sheer should be shunned.

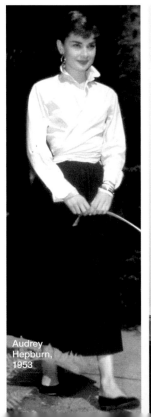

Audrey Hepburn, 1953

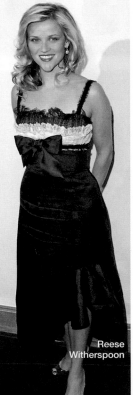

Reese Witherspoon

Grace Kelly, circa 1954

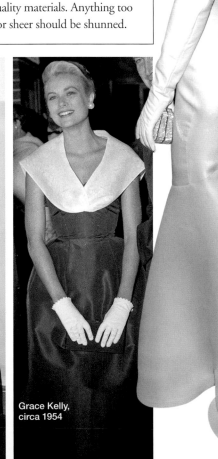

Renée Zellweger

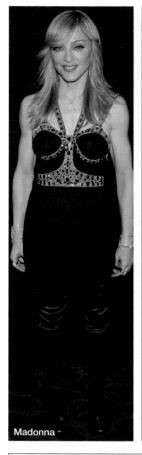

Madonna

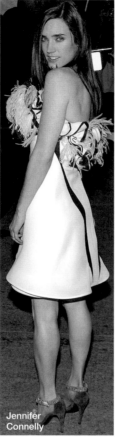

Jennifer Connelly

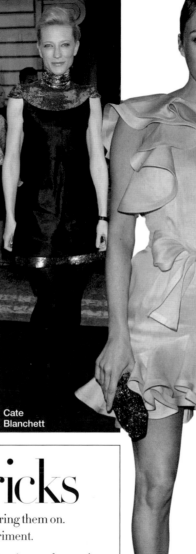

Cate Blanchett

Chloë Sevigny

The Mavericks

New designers? Avant-garde cuts? Bold looks? Bring them on.
This fashion-forward group is not afraid to experiment.

- **Don't follow the pack.** Look for pieces no one else has and start your own trends. (People will follow!)
- **Relish the unexpected.** The dress code calls for black tie? Try a short dress studded with sequins instead of the usual floor-length gown.
- **Seek out unique colors** and trimmings. Think taxicab yellow or marabou feathers.
- **To add just a slight edge** to your style, try working a supermodern accessory or two into your look.

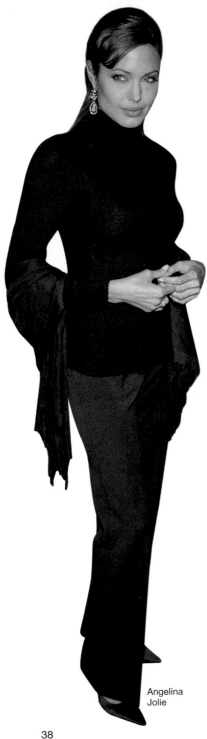

Angelina
Jolie

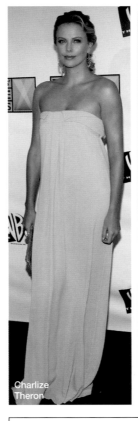

Charlize
Theron

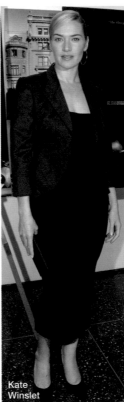

Kate
Winslet

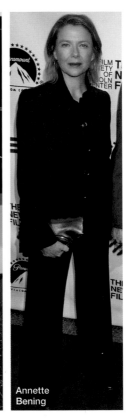

Annette
Bening

The Minimalists

Sleek, simple shapes in a monochrome, toned-down palette are what keep this clan looking sharp and smart

- **Black is your best friend.** The no-frills hue always works, whether in a skirt, top, pant, or dress.
- **Go for a lean line.** Clothes that are cut close to the body but aren't overtly sexy will serve you well.
- **Keep it reserved.** No need to be risqué or show too much skin.
- **Stay away from loud colors,** embellishments, and fanciful details. They aren't your thing.

The Eclectics

It's all about having fun with fashion for these playful women. Bright colors, madcap pairings, and loud patterns are part of the package.

- **Never say never.** Follow your heart when it comes to picking out your clothes. Forget what's appropriate or safe, and don't take yourself too seriously.
- **Eye-catching hues** and look-at-me motifs are par for the course.

- **Mixing and matching** makes sense. Try a tailored jacket over a funky frock, for example.
- **Be wary** of crossing the line into tackyville. Keep one piece pared down or your accessories classic when wearing something wacky.

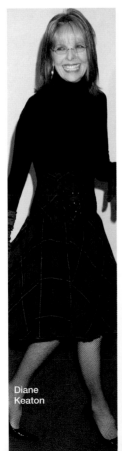

Diane Keaton

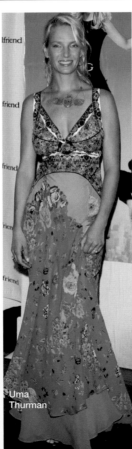

Uma Thurman

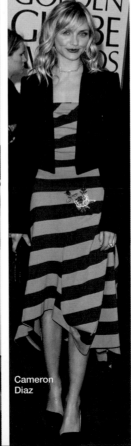

Cameron Diaz

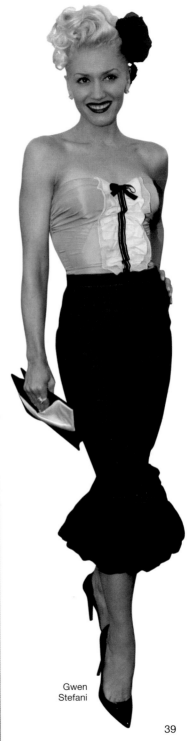

Gwen Stefani

Secrets of Stylish Women

The best-dressed women are exactly that because they wear the clothes and don't let the clothes wear them

Gwyneth Paltrow
Modern ✦ yet classic with a hint of cool

This fashion darling appreciates timeless essentials like jeans, blazers, and cardigans while embracing trends like minis, cropped pants, and raw-edged frocks. Paltrow effortlessly touches on the two sides of style and inevitably looks unpretentiously pulled together, down-to-earth, and utterly chic.

SHOWSTOPPER When it comes to entrances, it doesn't have to be about dripping beads or showing skin. Clearly, a covered-up, refined look can be just as glam. Pared-down gold jewelry and a red pout add to the elegance.

CASUAL For low-key looks, the actress keeps it basic with a little preppy appeal. The right combination of a T-shirt, shorts, and a sweater is an easy warm-weather go-to for day, and neutral tones keep it looking clean.

DRESSED-UP DAY Paltrow knows a shirtdress is the epitome of easy dressing. It works night and day, can be both sporty and sweet, and is always flattering. And she effortlessly mixes a classic bag with edgy boots.

COCKTAIL Big bows and sparkly details make every woman feel special. Paltrow picks a subtle palette and a cut that highlights the hourglass.

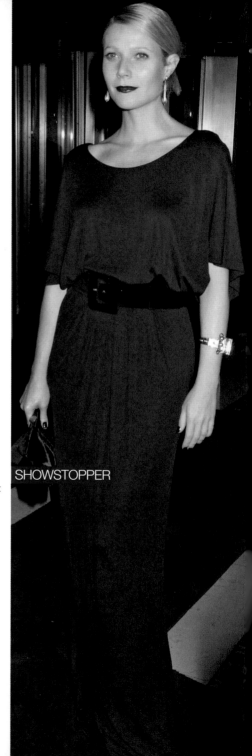

SHOWSTOPPER

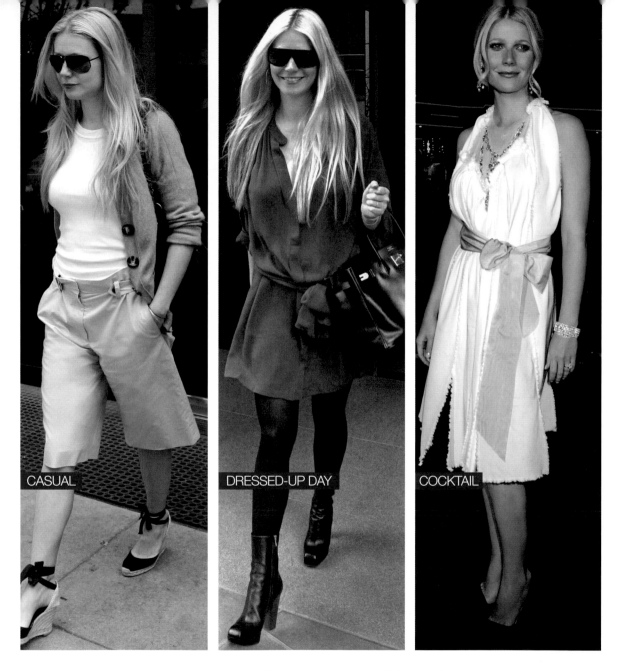

CASUAL

DRESSED-UP DAY

COCKTAIL

"My mother told me to **always dress like a lady** and I'd never regret it." —GWYNETH PALTROW

Sarah Jessica Parker

Quirky individualism is her fashion focus

The *Sex and the City* star loves clothes in all their forms. Never afraid to take chances, she deftly combines colors, textures, and shapes to add her unique élan to every outfit. Parker avoids getting stuck in that much-dreaded fashion rut and is consistent only about changing up her look, from modern and cool to boho babe to lovely lady.

SHOWSTOPPER Parker takes the red carpet in an überfeminine, retro-style frock, but it looks modern in the shocking green shade. Known for adding a personal touch to everything she wears, the actress boosts the dazzle factor with a deco brooch on her dress, with one in her hair as well.

CASUAL The jeans-and-a-jacket combo looks fresh when proportions are changed up, with a long, draped tee under a shorter topper. High-heel boots give a day look a sleeker, sexier edge.

DRESSED-UP DAY Parker is the master of mixing unexpected styles, like a jeweled tank with a tailored tweed jacket and a sweet dirndl. It makes for a fun day-to-night look. Lots of jewelry is a must.

COCKTAIL Never one for blending in with the crowds, the star forgoes the standard shift for something more sparkly and sexy—and doesn't hold back with a glam bag and shoes. But with such a standout dress and accessories, she opts for natural hair and goes jewelry free.

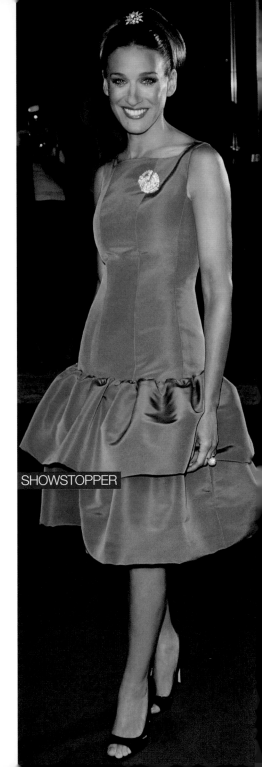

SHOWSTOPPER

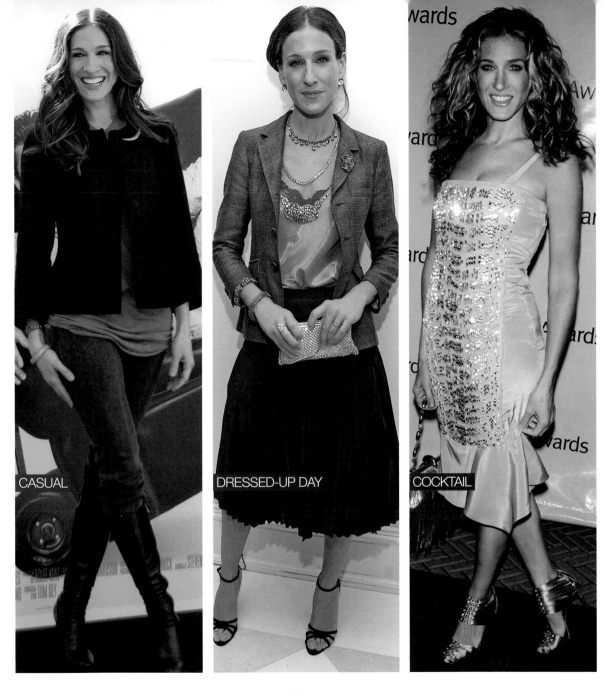

CASUAL

DRESSED-UP DAY

COCKTAIL

"I always think about my figure first." —SARAH JESSICA PARKER

Nicole Kidman

Elegant sophistication with a high-fashion flair

The Oscar winner never fails to present herself with polish and a bit of drama. While she certainly has access to designer clothes and pricey stylists, she clearly has honed her personal style. Kidman doesn't hesitate to experiment with edgier looks, she embraces femininity, and she often mixes in a dash of masculine inspiration with tailored jackets and pants. She's known for her mature and womanly dressing, choosing pieces that reflect her graceful demeanor.

SHOWSTOPPER For major galas, Kidman always shines. A regal-looking gold gown screams, "All eyes on me." She knows how to choose stunning numbers for the big nights.

CASUAL Kidman lets jeans take a tasteful turn and partners them with a ladylike blouse and a trim blazer. Leaner-cut denim also adds to the refinement of the look, and a sheer blouse lends a hint of sultriness.

DRESSED-UP DAY A pretty frock (that could also be perfect for evening) gets the daytime treatment when paired with black flats. The nipped waist on the flowy dress keeps it figure flattering.

COCKTAIL Sleek and sexy—but not overtly so—is Kidman's evening choice. A body-hugging number in a nearly nude shade with subtle sparkle is alluring, while the simple shape keeps it elegant.

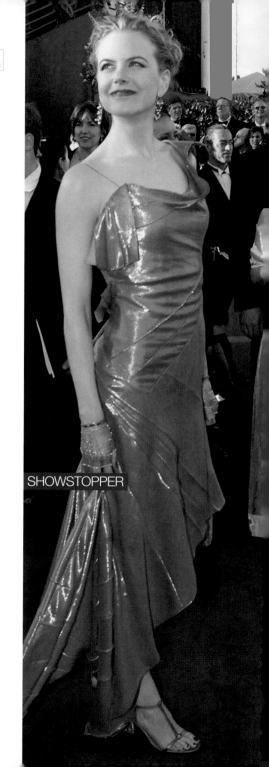

SHOWSTOPPER

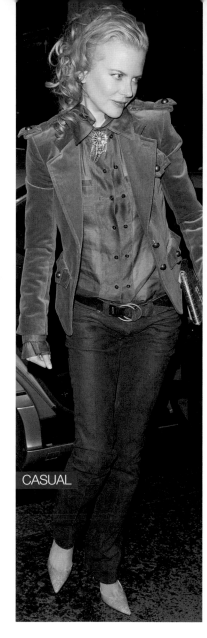

CASUAL

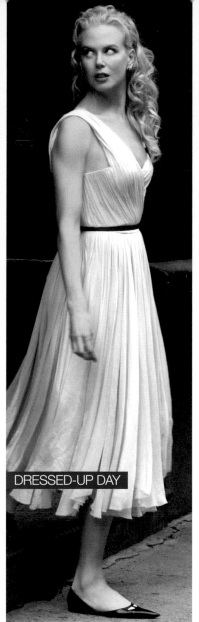

DRESSED-UP DAY

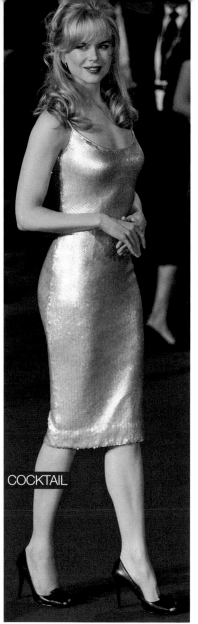

COCKTAIL

"I'm not big on very, very revealing clothes. If I show a bit of skin in one place, I'll cover the rest. I'm not a big fan of cleavage— not that I have a lot of cleavage! It's not my thing." —NICOLE KIDMAN

Demi Moore

Flirty and fun but fashion forward is her mantra

She's a gorgeous brunette with a killer body, and she's consistently glamorous, everywhere from the red carpet to a city street. Moore's style is modern—she's usually in the latest designer looks—but never forced or too trendy. She makes every piece chic. Whether it's showing off her great legs or highlighting her trim waist, she also knows how to make the most of her figure.

SHOWSTOPPER A gorgeous color, a rich mix of fabrics, a hint of lace, fishnets, and a bow—Moore's got the perfect combination for a stunning look. And she proves that showing a bit of lingerie isn't tarty when your outfit is so chic.

CASUAL Let's just say it's all relative. A more low-key look for Moore still has a major glam factor. But it's about balance: A glossy, metallic top is the ideal match for worn-in denim because the sexy shirt is toned down by the basic jeans.

DRESSED-UP DAY A simple dress couldn't be easier to throw on. A solid, sober shade like gray gives it the ability to work well for night, and a waist cincher gives it a flattering line.

COCKTAIL If you've got great gams, go ahead and show them off in a shorter frock. A unique cut, à la the bubble hem, and an interesting hue, like ombre grays and greens, keep a leggy look from seeming too youthful. And again, a wide belt makes a voluminous silhouette more body conscious.

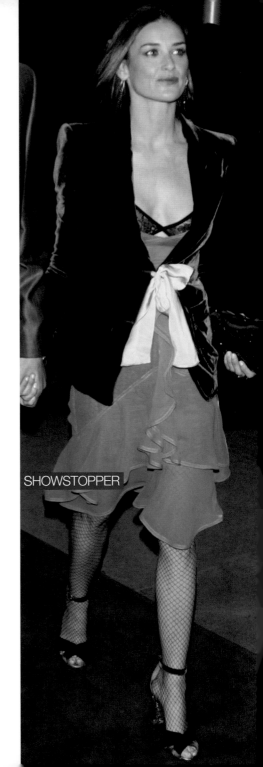

SHOWSTOPPER

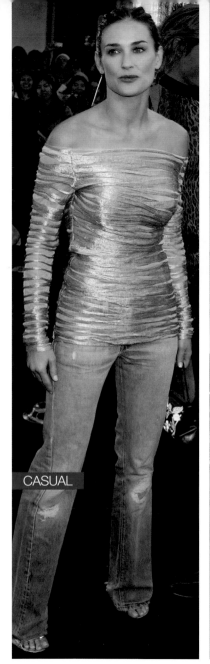

CASUAL

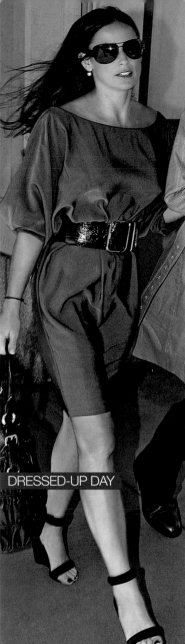

DRESSED-UP DAY

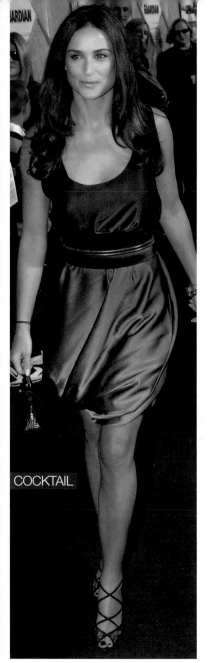

COCKTAIL

"Whether a piece was \$5,000 or \$5,
I can love it the same." —DEMI MOORE

Expert Advice

What a designer can teach you about finding your own style

Carolina Herrera

The Venezuelan style arbiter is all about class, elegance, and ladylike refinement. Women turn to her for polished separates and gowns—and when they do, they're guaranteed to look sophisticated.

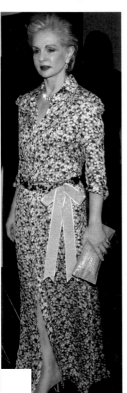

PERSONAL STYLE IS…
Not only about the clothes. It is about knowledge, manners, the way one moves, talks, and wears the clothes that make it personal for oneself.

HOW TO FIND IT:
Women can find their personal style by ignoring trends and choosing classic, timeless pieces.

TRIED-AND-TRUE FASHION TIPS:
Wear the right styles for your age and your figure. And always keep in mind the occasion that you are dressing for.

Diane von Furstenberg

She made a sensation with the invention of the all-purpose wrap dress, giving women an easy day-to-night option. This jet-setter epitomizes what her clothes are about: effortless polish for women on the go.

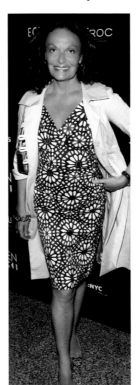

PERSONAL STYLE IS…
Accepting who you are and then going with it—which means know who you are, what you like, and what your assets are.

HOW TO FIND IT:
Keep an elastic body and an elastic mind, and be as flexible as you can. And just enjoy life.

TRIED-AND-TRUE FASHION TIPS:
Pick things you are comfortable in. If you feel well within yourself, within your skin, then you will look more confident—and if you look more confident, you look more beautiful.

Donna Karan

Her "seven easy pieces" revolutionized the working woman's wardrobe, and she's all about not sacrificing comfort for chic. The result is cool, urban clothes that feel as good as they look.

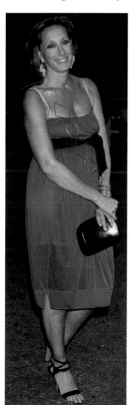

PERSONAL STYLE IS…
What you are comfortable with, what you relate to. My personal style is sensual, comfortable, black, day to night.

SECRET TO STYLE:
Simplicity—the less-is-more theory. Start with a basic foundation and build upon that. Style comes from within, and if you stay true to yourself, you have style.

TRIED-AND-TRUE FASHION TIPS:
Dress for your own individual spirit and lifestyle. That matters much more than what's in or out of fashion in a given moment. The most important fashion tip I can give is this: Wear what you feel good in and don't let the clothes wear you.

Donatella Versace

This Italian fashion diva amps up the sex appeal and takes glamour to the highest level. She offers women curve-hugging, strut-your-stuff fashion that's for the bold and daring.

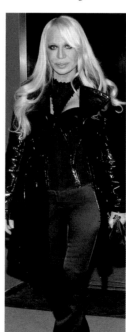

PERSONAL STYLE IS…
Confidence.

HOW TO FIND IT:
Listen to your inner voice. First instincts are usually the right ones. Choose items that you feel comfortable wearing, and don't be afraid to try new things. Most important, feel good about what you're wearing.

SECRET TO STYLE:
Choose a wardrobe that reflects your lifestyle, your passions, and your dreams.

TRIED-AND-TRUE FASHION TIPS:
Never follow a trend just because it's a trend. If you feel sensual, confident, and glamorous, chances are you are very much in vogue.

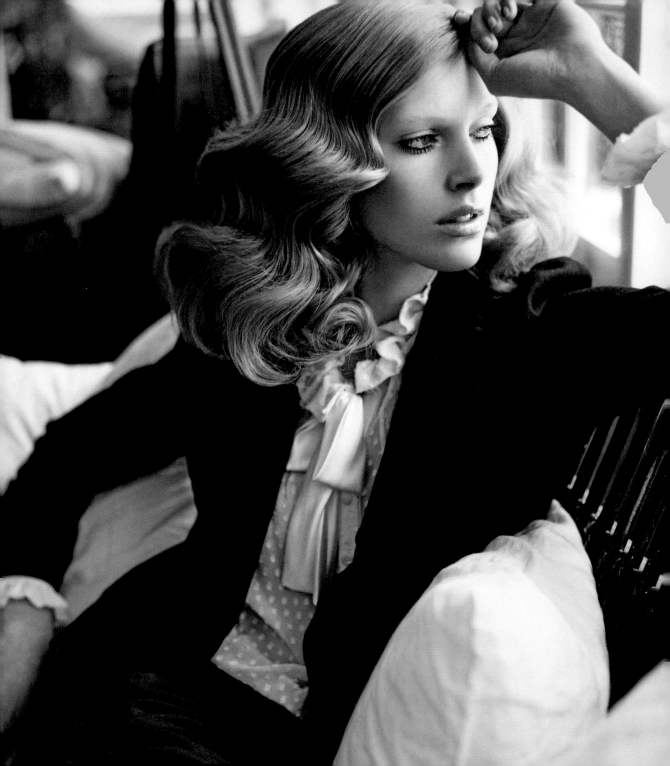

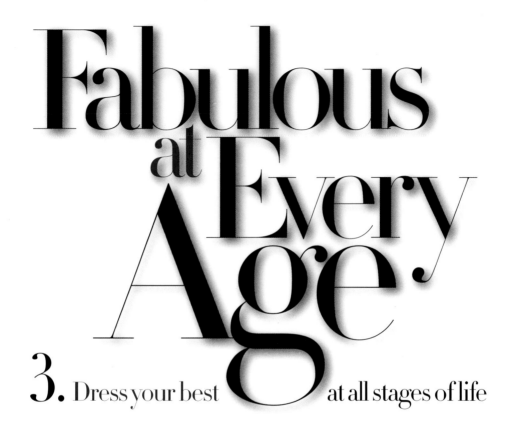

Fabulous at Every Age

3. Dress your best at all stages of life

"Zest is the secret of all beauty. There is no beauty that is attractive without zest."
——CHRISTIAN DIOR

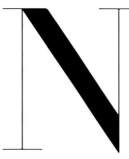

No doubt these thoughts have gone through your mind when you've stood in front of the mirror: Am I dressing like my mother? Do I look like I'm wearing my daughter's clothes? Am I dressing age appropriately? Am I making the most of my looks? Perhaps your frock is in an eye-popping color or print, skims the body, plunges low in front or back, or shows too much skin. Maybe it doesn't show enough skin and adds years. And with all the boundary breaking in fashion today, it is not always clear who should wear what.

First and foremost, style is about inner confidence. If you are 50 and dare to wear a mini, more power to you. (However, be prepared for heads to turn and eyebrows to raise if you don't get it right.) If you tend to err on the safe side but still like to be in the fashion game, there are plenty of interesting and chic options out there for you, no matter what your age. From "anything goes" in your 20s to toned-down hues and sculpted cuts in your 40s to luxe fabrics in your 70s, find out what's best for you and you'll always look and feel poised in your clothes.

What to consider when dressing for your age:

20s **There are no boundaries** for twentysomethings when it comes to fashion. It's about personal style and adding whimsical touches you can get away with only when you're young, whether that means playing with color, mixing and matching, or wearing high heels and high hemlines.

30s **More pulled-together, serious looks** are what your 30s are about, but you don't have to be a total square. The trick is to experiment with fashion-forward styles while maintaining a level of polish.

40s **Classic silhouettes and colors** may start to dominate your wardrobe, but each piece should be full of personality. Think interesting embellishment, feminine volume, and bursts of rich color and pattern.

50s **Refined, tasteful choices** are the foundations of age-appropriate dressing. Tailoring and structure are key, as are clean lines and fuss-free pieces in a simple palette.

60s **Elegance is the idea,** and so timeless, traditional pieces are the mainstays. Tweed suits, trousers, and coatdresses dominate the closet. Contrasting hues—black, white, and red—are the most chic.

70+ **Looking dignified and distinguished** is of the utmost importance—and that means splurging on a little luxury. Fabrics should be of the highest quality, and tailoring should be precise.

> "Age is but a number! Wear what you like and love what you wear! Forget your age!" —KATE HUDSON

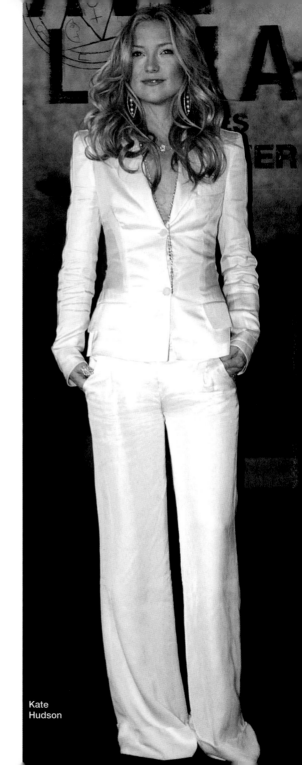

Kate
Hudson

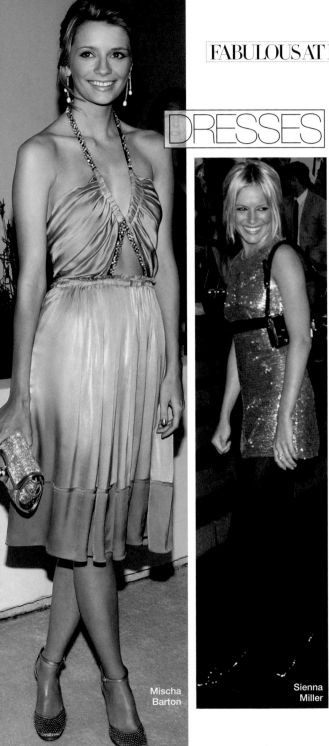
Mischa
Barton

DRESSES

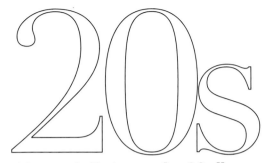
Sienna
Miller

20s

Ah, youth. Being under 30 allows you to get away with a lot when it comes to dressing.

- **Pick a fun frock.** Ultrafeminine, lighthearted, colorful, and flirty are the qualities to look for in a dress, whether it's for night or day. Don't be afraid to show a little skin here and there, but remember to maintain a level of polish. If your dress is revealing on top, make sure the hemline is a little longer. If it's short, the silhouette should be more restrained.

- **Try a top with personality.** It could have loads of ruffles, highlight your décolletage in a strapless cut, or even be a washed-out rocker tee—as long as it's interesting. We all know the youthful set loves jeans, which go with every sort of shirt and blouse, so let your top set the tone for your look.

- **When it comes to skirts, think sweet or sexy.** Twentysomethings can pull off charming pouf, pleated, and bubble-hemmed skirts. If you have the body for it, go for minis, tight or full. Either way, your top should be toned down when your skirt is special.

- **Experiment with jackets and coats.** Wear a tailored blazer over a floaty frock, a sleek leather bomber with a breezy, floral blouse, or a girly, princess-cut coat atop skinny jeans and a tank.

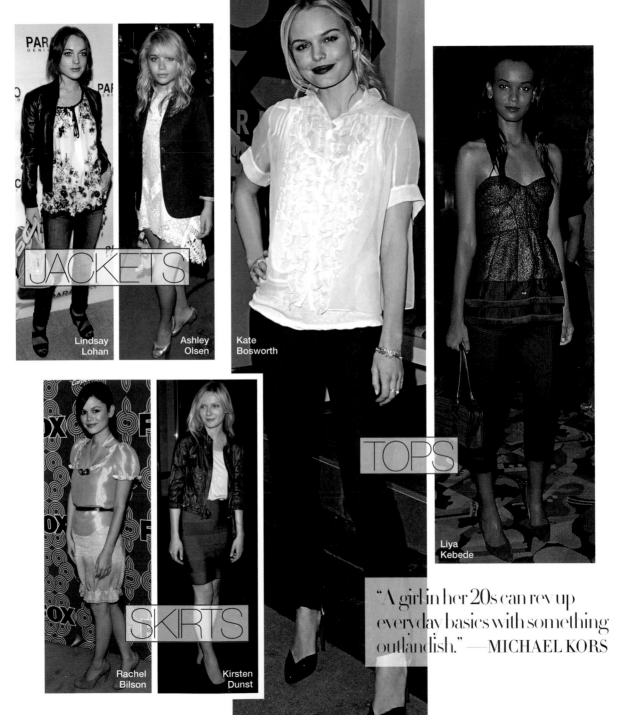

JACKETS

Lindsay Lohan

Ashley Olsen

Kate Bosworth

TOPS

Liya Kebede

SKIRTS

Rachel Bilson

Kirsten Dunst

"A girl in her 20s can rev up everyday basics with something outlandish." —MICHAEL KORS

GET THE LOOK

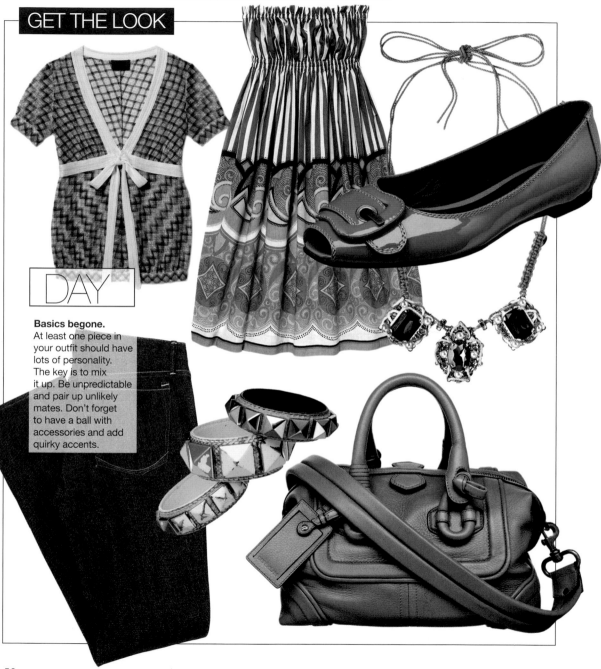

DAY

Basics begone.
At least one piece in your outfit should have lots of personality. The key is to mix it up. Be unpredictable and pair up unlikely mates. Don't forget to have a ball with accessories and add quirky accents.

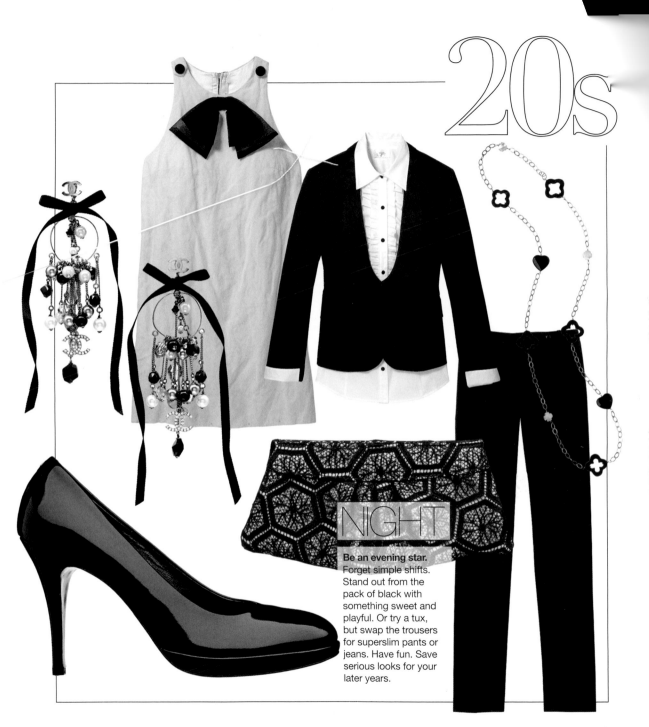

NIGHT

Be an evening star. Forget simple shifts. Stand out from the pack of black with something sweet and playful. Or try a tux, but swap the trousers for superslim pants or jeans. Have fun. Save serious looks for your later years.

JACKETS

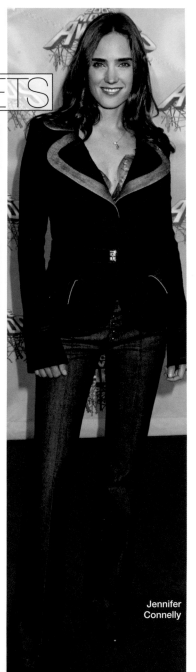

Gwen
Stefani

COATS

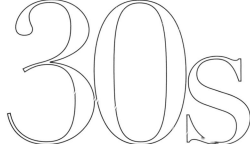

30s

A honed sense of style leads to sophistication, but don't put your risk-taking days behind

- **Go for a dress in a new silhouette.** Whether it's below the knee or well above, revealing, roomy, or in between, pick a shape that's interesting and unique. Try contrasting shades, metallics, and pops of brights. The idea is to look cool and confident. Move beyond the superslinky and girly stuff.

- **Your shirt should have an edge.** It can be a crisp button-up, a silk blouse, or a simple tee, but it should have a fresh twist. Neat ruffles, a prim scarf tie, or a bit of ruching can turn a basic into something bold.

- **Seek out skirts with style.** Though it's a feminine signature, a skirt doesn't have to be mumsy. Look for pieces that are either sharp and severe or soft and subtle. A sculpted pencil shape with a high waist is seriously sophisticated but not stuffy, while a swingy, short skirt adds attitude.

- **Top off your look with something striking.** Your coat or jacket is an integral part of your wardrobe, so pick a piece that makes a statement. A trim, architectural jacket can be just as dramatic as a bold animal-print coat.

Jennifer
Connelly

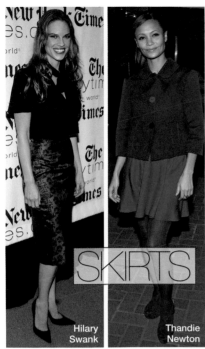

SKIRTS

Hilary Swank

Thandie Newton

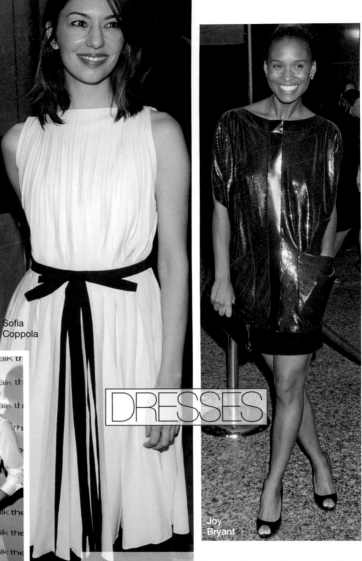

Sofia Coppola

DRESSES

Joy Bryant

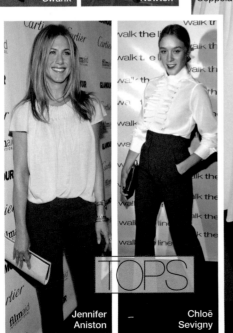

TOPS

Jennifer Aniston

Chloë Sevigny

"I don't know if I really understand the idea of dressing for one's age. All you need is confidence, comfort, and the pleasure of dressing." —MARC JACOBS

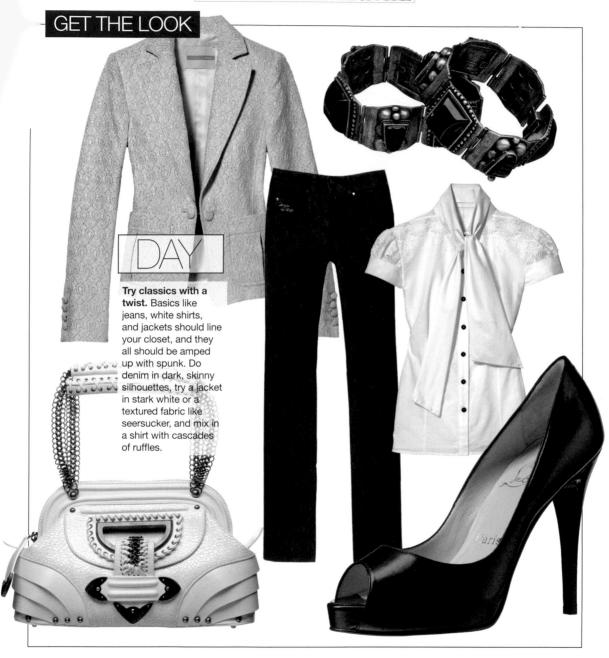

DAY

Try classics with a twist. Basics like jeans, white shirts, and jackets should line your closet, and they all should be amped up with spunk. Do denim in dark, skinny silhouettes, try a jacket in stark white or a textured fabric like seersucker, and mix in a shirt with cascades of ruffles.

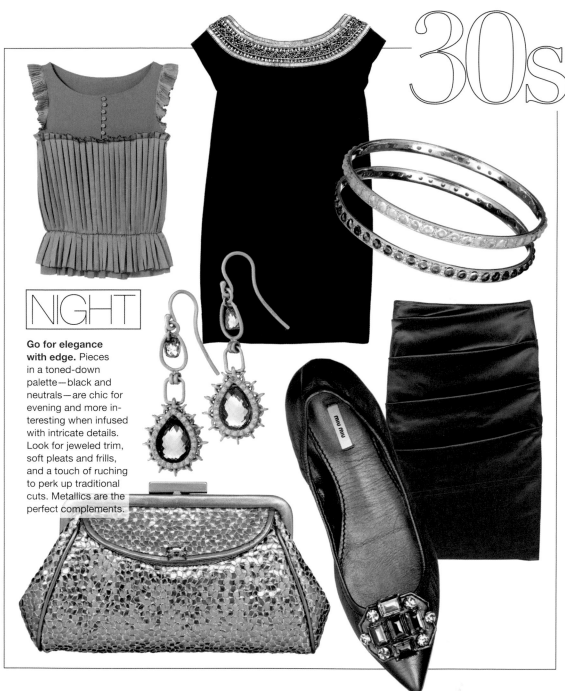

NIGHT

Go for elegance with edge. Pieces in a toned-down palette—black and neutrals—are chic for evening and more interesting when infused with intricate details. Look for jeweled trim, soft pleats and frills, and a touch of ruching to perk up traditional cuts. Metallics are the perfect complements.

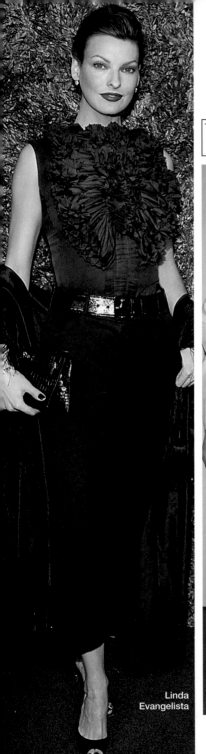

Linda
Evangelista

TOPS

40s

It's important to look smart and conservative, but that doesn't have to mean buttoned up

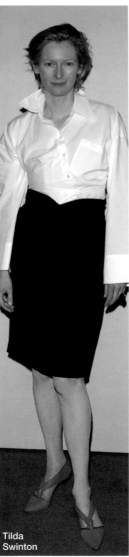

Tilda
Swinton

- **Find a refined frock.** You want a mature but not matronly look. More covered-up cuts that fall at the knee or just below are appropriate, but there are plenty of pieces that still have sex appeal. A formfitting shape, cinched-in waist, or strategic cutouts will do the trick.

- **Opt for a subdued yet modern top.** It's a no-brainer: A stark shirt is überversatile and universally flattering. Something more complex, however, like a frothy, frilled piece, can be an outfit maker. But choose wisely; when going for something with detail, pick a solid, sophisticated shade.

- **Stick to fine and feminine skirts.** Demonstrate more restraint when it comes to showing leg—but not necessarily with your skirt style. A full, pleated cut looks sweet and womanly, while a below-the-knee pencil is a sleek standard. Also, fancy details on a skirt give your look an interesting, high-quality air.

- **Consider a well-constructed jacket cut.** Whether it's to be worn with jeans or a dress, your blazer or coat should have structure. Shapes that emphasize the hourglass look stylized and sophisticated. A roomier, boxier cut will easily go over any outfit.

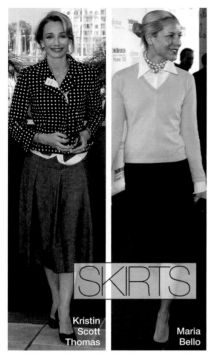

SKIRTS

Kristin Scott Thomas

Maria Bello

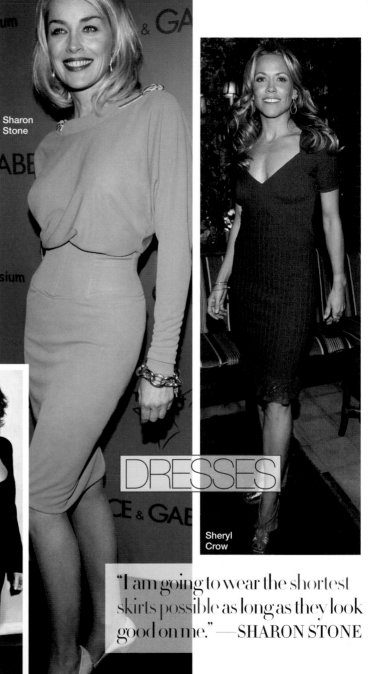

Sharon Stone

DRESSES

Sheryl Crow

"I am going to wear the shortest skirts possible as long as they look good on me." —SHARON STONE

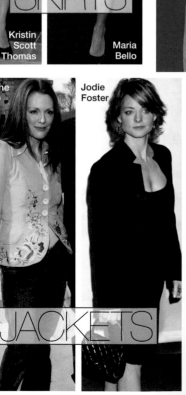

Julianne Moore

Jodie Foster

JACKETS

GET THE LOOK

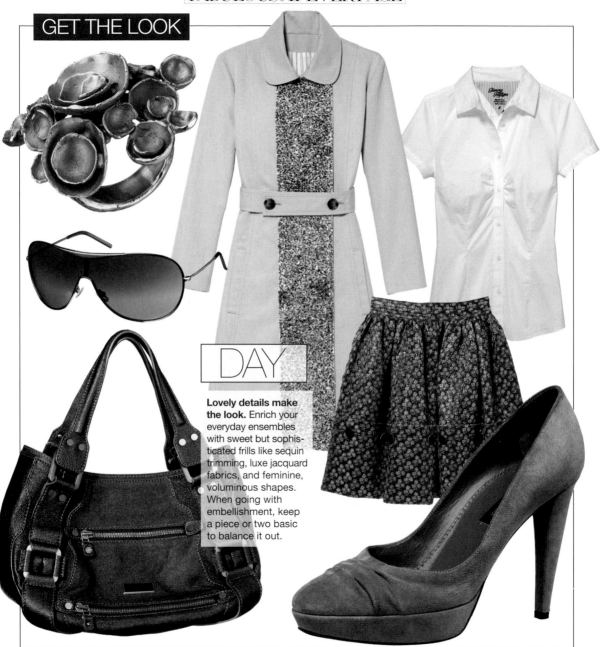

DAY

Lovely details make the look. Enrich your everyday ensembles with sweet but sophisticated frills like sequin trimming, luxe jacquard fabrics, and feminine, voluminous shapes. When going with embellishment, keep a piece or two basic to balance it out.

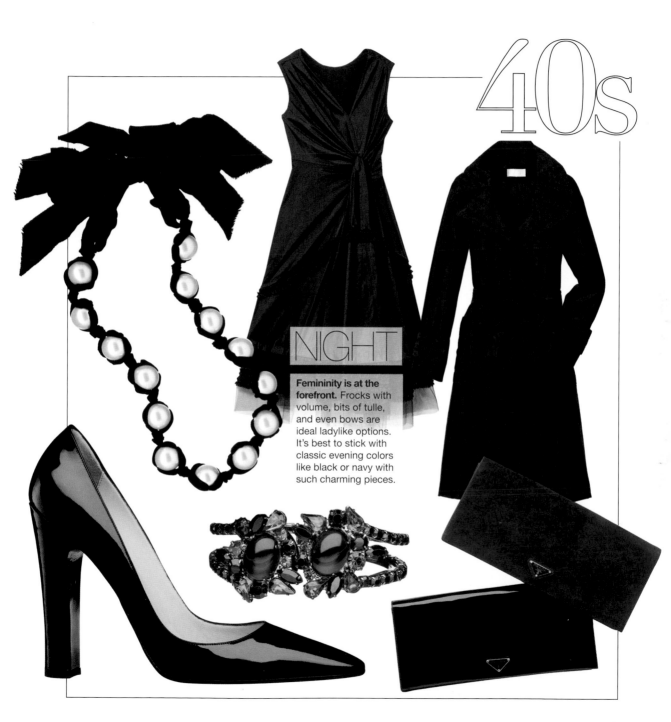

40s

NIGHT

Femininity is at the forefront. Frocks with volume, bits of tulle, and even bows are ideal ladylike options. It's best to stick with classic evening colors like black or navy with such charming pieces.

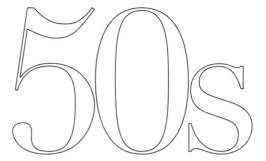

50s

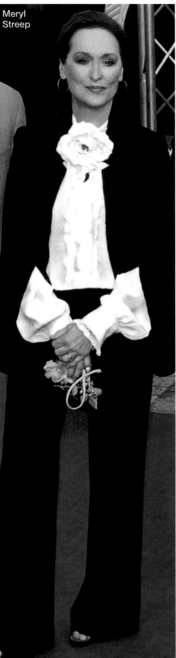

Meryl Streep

TOPS

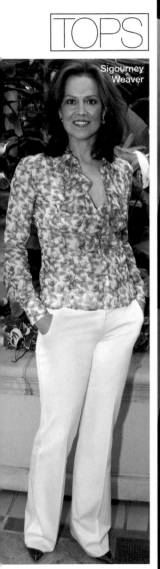

Sigourney Weaver

Now is the time to embrace traditional elegance with uptown appeal. Leave the latest trends by the wayside.

- **Dress up in classic colors.** Choose solids in lush but low-key shades; deep brown, navy, and black look best. This, however, does not mean boring. Go for cuts with interesting and complex details like accordion pleats or a gathered waist.

- **Look for ladylike tops.** Billowing, blousy tops—like scarf-tie, ruffle-front, or full-sleeved styles—give a soft edge to more structured separates. When a top has lots of volume, however, the color or print should be muted, as should your bottoms.

- **Keep your skirt simple or luxe it up.** A long, lean cut is classic—and the perfect accompaniment to your flouncier tops. But a slightly sexy, playful style, cut in lace or adorned with ruffles, is a fun alternative when paired with something basic. And keep the hemline in check.

- **Start with a clean-cut jacket.** A sleek blazer will go with everything and go anywhere. Add sumptuous styles like a short fur or embellished topper to your wardrobe for evenings out or just to glam it up for day.

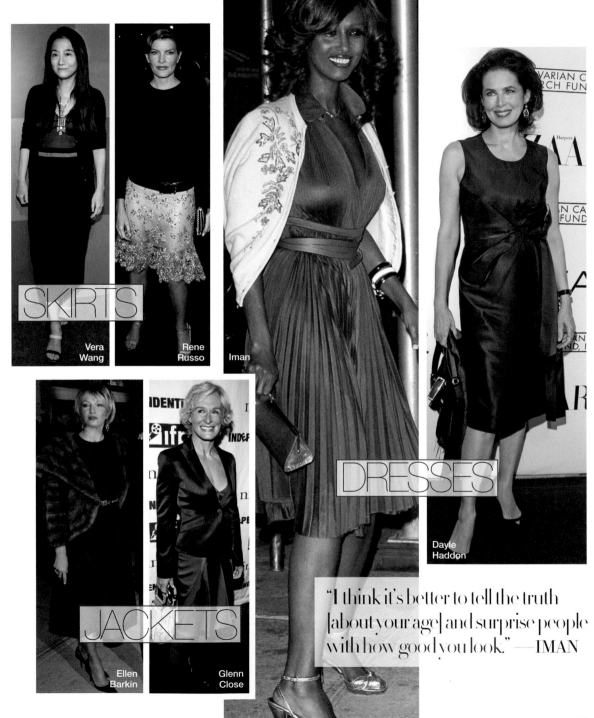

SKIRTS

Vera Wang

Rene Russo

Iman

DRESSES

Dayle Haddon

JACKETS

Ellen Barkin

Glenn Close

"I think it's better to tell the truth [about your age] and surprise people with how good you look." —IMAN

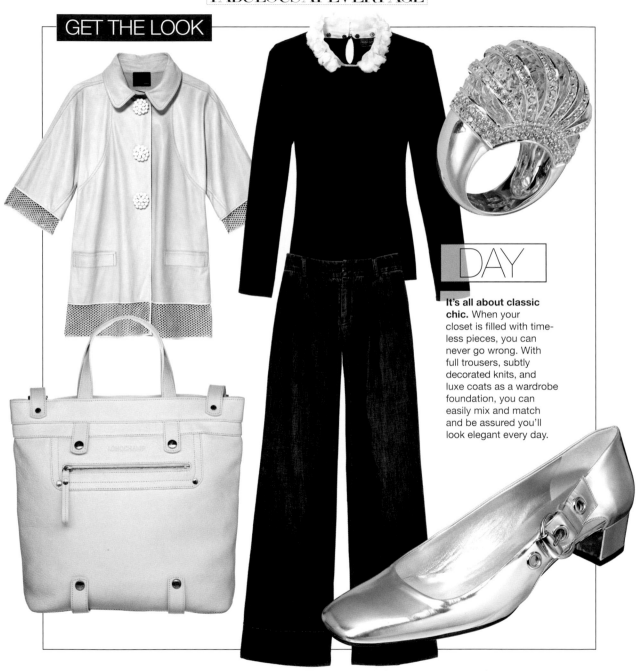

GET THE LOOK

DAY

It's all about classic chic. When your closet is filled with timeless pieces, you can never go wrong. With full trousers, subtly decorated knits, and luxe coats as a wardrobe foundation, you can easily mix and match and be assured you'll look elegant every day.

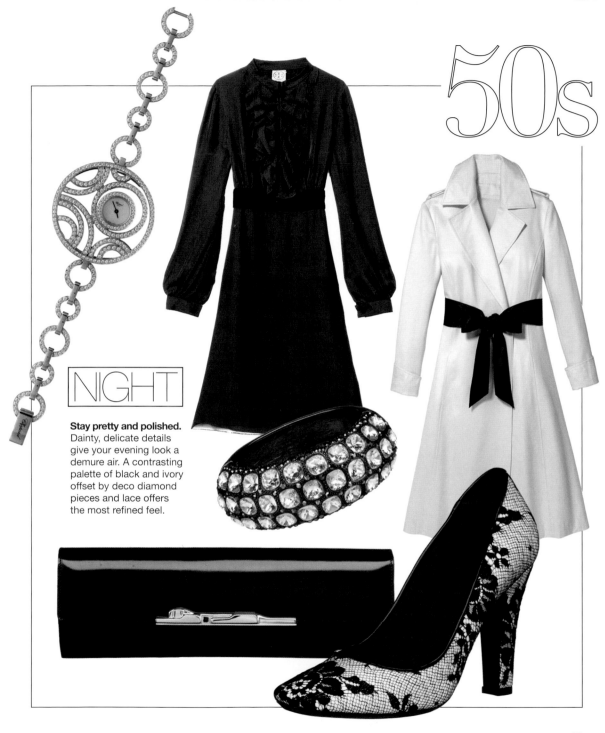

50s

NIGHT

Stay pretty and polished.
Dainty, delicate details give your evening look a demure air. A contrasting palette of black and ivory offset by deco diamond pieces and lace offers the most refined feel.

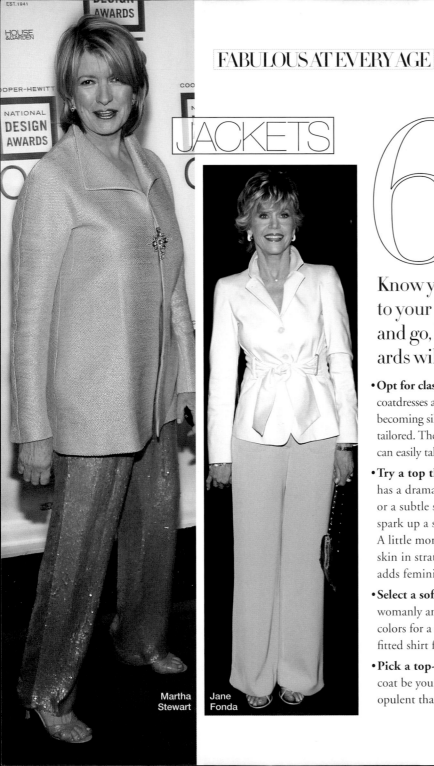

JACKETS

60s

Know your style and be true to your instincts. Fads come and go, but enduring standards will serve you well.

- **Opt for classic-cut dresses.** Shirtdresses and coatdresses are mainstays. They provide a becoming silhouette, and structure keeps them tailored. They also offer endless options. You can easily take these frocks from day to night.

- **Try a top that's eye-catching.** Whether it has a dramatic detail like overblown frills or a subtle sheen from gold satin, it should spark up a suit or a simple skirt or trouser. A little more coverage is key, but showing skin in strategic places like the décolletage adds femininity.

- **Select a soft skirt.** A swingy A-line shape is womanly and flattering, and go with solid colors for a cleaner look. Pair it with a more fitted shirt for just the right balance.

- **Pick a top-notch topper.** Let a jacket or coat be your centerpiece. Look for something opulent that still retains a certain timelessness.

Martha Stewart

Jane Fonda

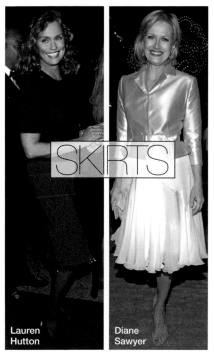

SKIRTS

Lauren
Hutton

Diane
Sawyer

Blythe
Danner

TOPS

Marisa
Berenson

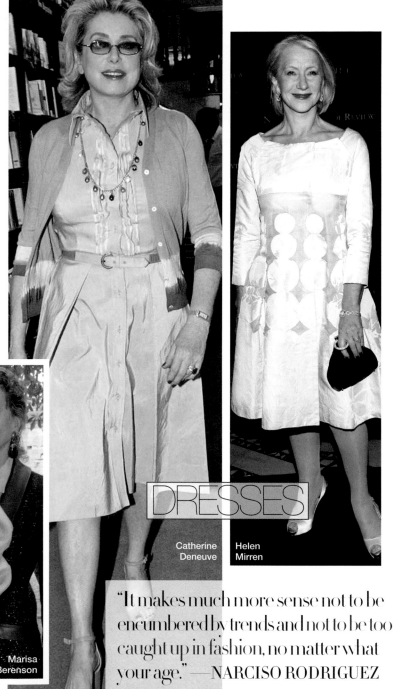

DRESSES

Catherine
Deneuve

Helen
Mirren

"It makes much more sense not to be encumbered by trends and not to be too caught up in fashion, no matter what your age." —NARCISO RODRIGUEZ

GET THE LOOK

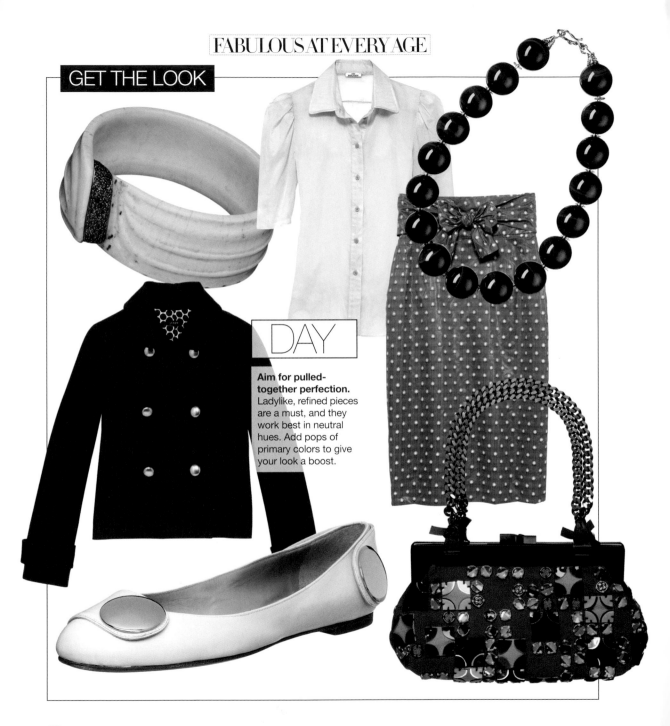

DAY

Aim for pulled-together perfection. Ladylike, refined pieces are a must, and they work best in neutral hues. Add pops of primary colors to give your look a boost.

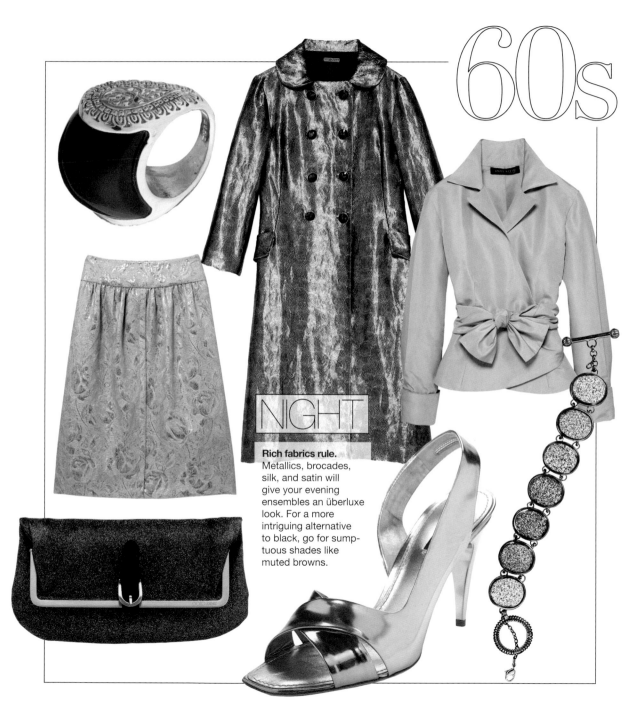

NIGHT

Rich fabrics rule.
Metallics, brocades, silk, and satin will give your evening ensembles an überluxe look. For a more intriguing alternative to black, go for sumptuous shades like muted browns.

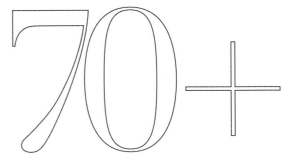

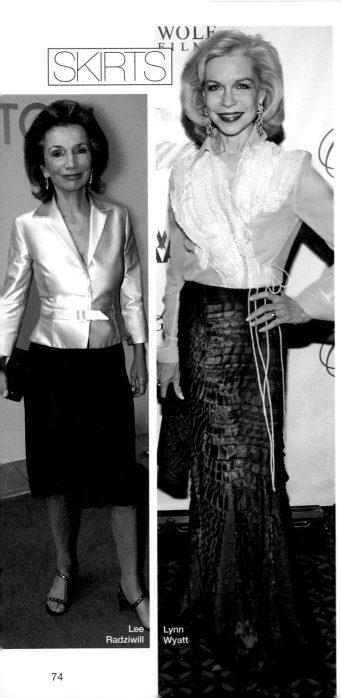

SKIRTS

Lee
Radziwill

Lynn
Wyatt

70+

Stay true to timeless, tailored shapes, but add lushness to your look with embellished pieces. Classic hues will ensure the utmost elegance.

- **Turn up the volume on top.** A gorgeous blouse can turn any look into a luxurious one. If it's in a muted tone, don't worry about going all the way with frills, ruffles, and lace.

- **A structured suit is standard.** Consider plush tones of ivory, chocolate, and beige your new neutrals. Of course, black is a given. A shape with a nipped-in waist is most becoming.

- **Go to great lengths for the perfect skirt.** Hemlines count, and styles that are below the knee for day and sweep the floor for night are ideal. Dark shades offer a more streamlined look.

- **Jackets and coats should be standouts.** A great one can be the focus of your look. Look for exquisite tailoring and quality fabrics. For a slim line, pass up the big prints; solids are more complementary.

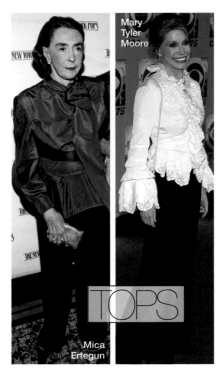

Mica Ertegun

Mary Tyler Moore

TOPS

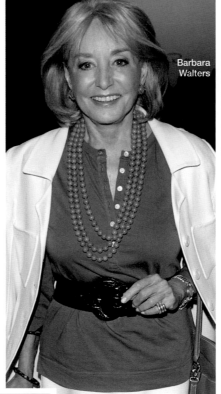

Barbara Walters

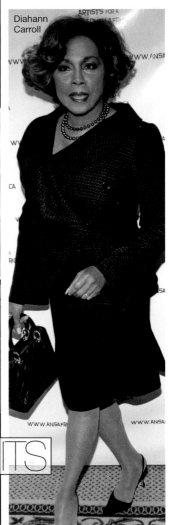

Diahann Carroll

SUITS

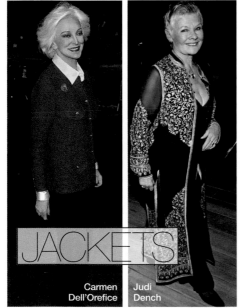

JACKETS

Carmen Dell'Orefice

Judi Dench

"I think an older woman can be more fascinating than a younger one. Dress elegantly and you will possess timeless and ageless style." — GIORGIO ARMANI

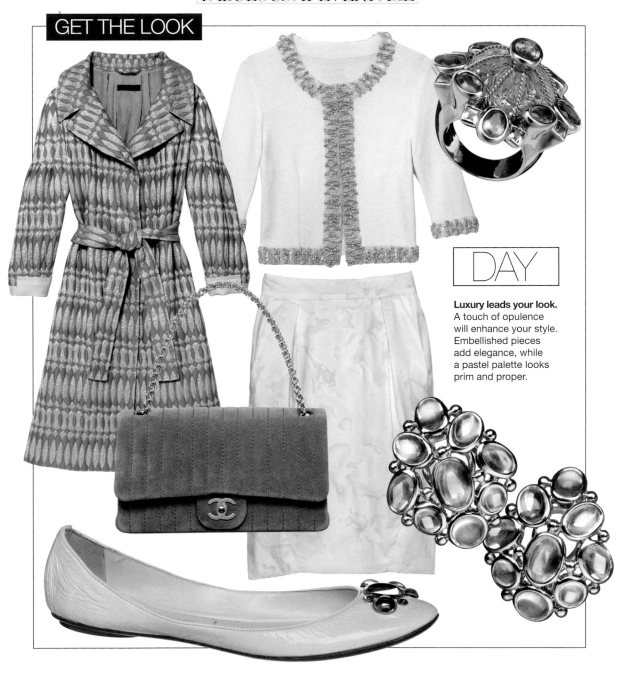

GET THE LOOK

DAY

Luxury leads your look.
A touch of opulence
will enhance your style.
Embellished pieces
add elegance, while
a pastel palette looks
prim and proper.

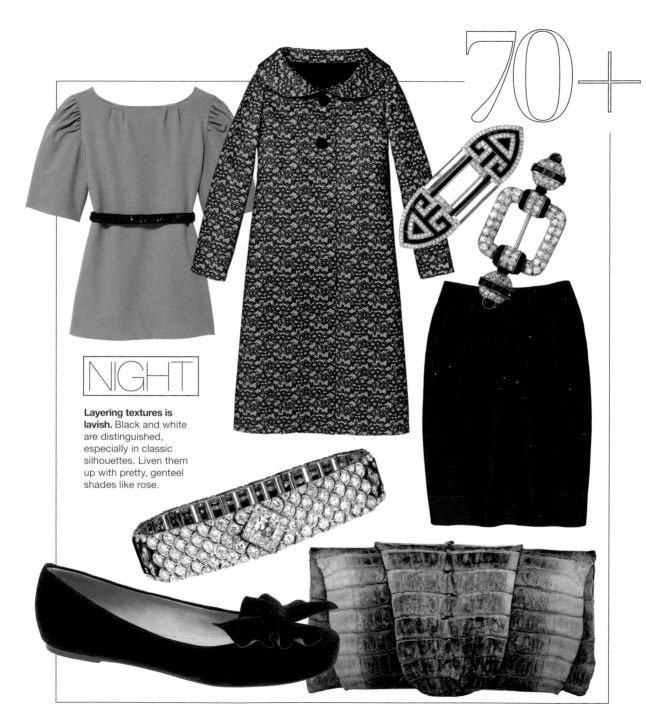

NIGHT

Layering textures is lavish. Black and white are distinguished, especially in classic silhouettes. Liven them up with pretty, genteel shades like rose.

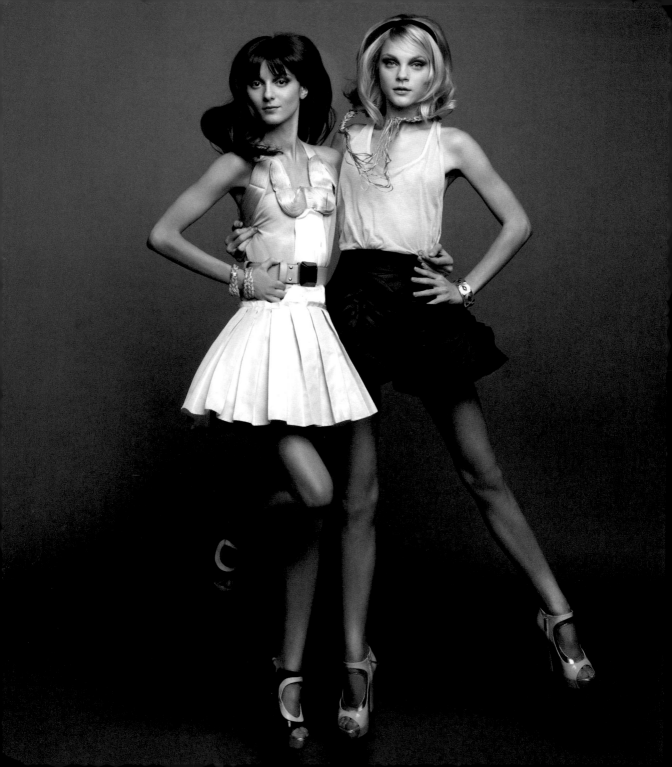

Celebrate Your Shape

4. Know how to flatter your figure

"I have never known a really chic woman whose **appearance** was not, in large part, an outward reflection of **her inner self.**"
—MAINBOCHER

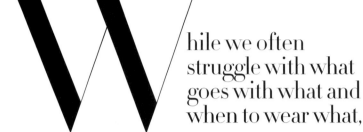

While we often struggle with what goes with what and when to wear what, let's be honest: The biggest question we most often ask ourselves is "Does this make me look fat?" We've all had many I-don't-want-to-leave-the-house moments when nothing seems to fit and nothing seems to look right. Yes, dressing for one's body is challenging for everyone. Whether you're thin, tall, or short or have broad shoulders, narrow shoulders, a flat butt, a round butt, no hips, or big hips, you probably have some body issues you are concerned with when it comes to finding clothes that fit. But this definitely should not be the cause of distress, as there are many ways to conquer these difficulties. The starting point is being honest with yourself and then accepting who you are. Embrace your figure. Celebrate it! Allow clothing to be your ally, not the enemy. With a little consideration and some strategy, you can use your clothes to flatter your figure, always.

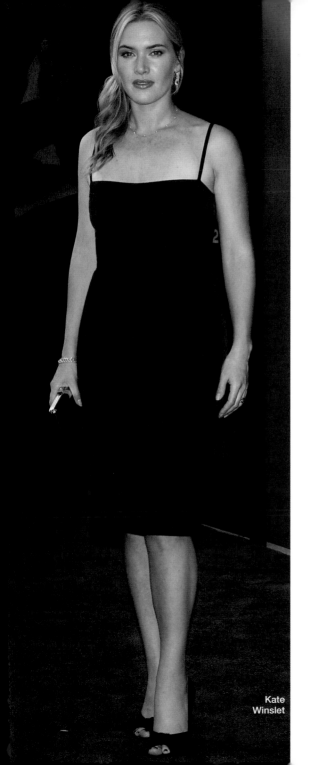

Kate
Winslet

What to consider when learning to dress best for your figure:

1. **Look in the mirror** and make an honest assessment of your body. Embrace your shape and who you are.

2. **Know your assets**—whether it's well-sculpted arms, a swanlike neck, or a wasp waist—and dress to enhance those features.

3. **Accept the parts** you are less than thrilled with and dress to de-emphasize them.

4. **Consider the pieces** you feel most comfortable in. Dresses? Trousers? Jeans? Button-ups? Sweaters? Then focus on finding the best cuts for you.

5. **Be open to experimenting** with new silhouettes. Pieces you've always shunned could end up being the most flattering.

"I just look better in simple black things."
—KATE WINSLET

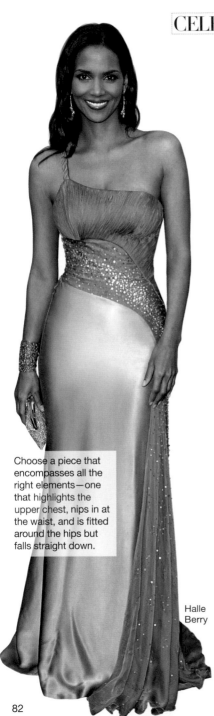

Choose a piece that encompasses all the right elements—one that highlights the upper chest, nips in at the waist, and is fitted around the hips but falls straight down.

Halle Berry

Curvy

Feminine clothes that enhance the hourglass are always flattering

- **Go trim.** To accentuate your figure, wear formfitting dresses and skirts that are cut diagonally or on the bias. They should nip in at the waist, hug the hips, and fall loosely over the thighs and calves.
- **Try it tailored.** A-line shapes will downplay your lower half. Choose structured pieces with a flare that isn't too dramatic; an exaggerated trapeze shape won't do you any favors. Whatever you wear on top, make sure it's slim and cut close to the body to best balance a fuller-cut lower half.
- **Work the middle.** Your waist should always be well defined. A cinched-in midriff never fails to flatter; it highlights your womanly figure. Wear a belt or choose pieces with details like beading or ruching at the waist.
- **Show skin—on top or bottom.** Be tactical about where it is revealed. A slit on the side of a gown can be sexy and slimming, while showing lots of leg offers a long, lean look. Highlighting your décolletage also looks sultry without being too provocative.
- **Select solid shades and color-blocking.** A tonal look proves to be a winning choice. Black is always flattering, but that doesn't mean color should be avoided. Add bits of brights in the right places, mix and match solids, and avoid eye-popping patterns. Simple shades like neutral brown, black, and navy look best.

"If I don't feel like it looks good on my body, I'm not going to wear it." —HALLE BERRY

82

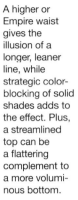

A higher or Empire waist gives the illusion of a longer, leaner line, while strategic color-blocking of solid shades adds to the effect. Plus, a streamlined top can be a flattering complement to a more voluminous bottom.

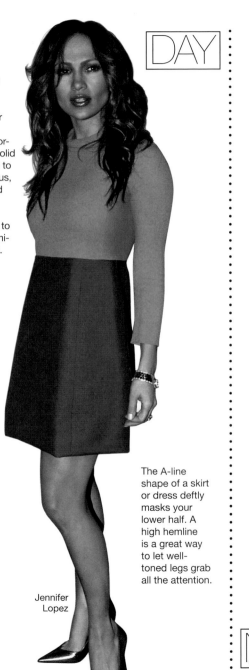

The A-line shape of a skirt or dress deftly masks your lower half. A high hemline is a great way to let well-toned legs grab all the attention.

Jennifer Lopez

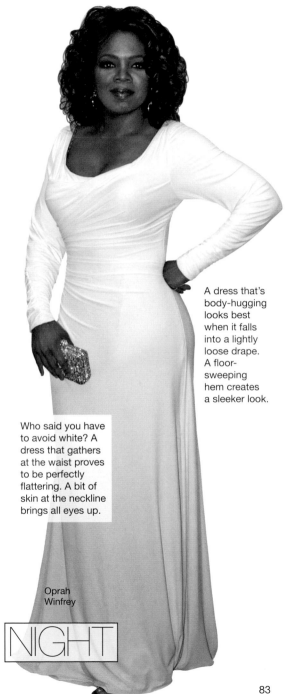

A dress that's body-hugging looks best when it falls into a lightly loose drape. A floor-sweeping hem creates a sleeker look.

Who said you have to avoid white? A dress that gathers at the waist proves to be perfectly flattering. A bit of skin at the neckline brings all eyes up.

Oprah Winfrey

NIGHT

83

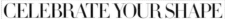

Fuller Figured

Consider simplicity, subtle sexiness, and a little structure

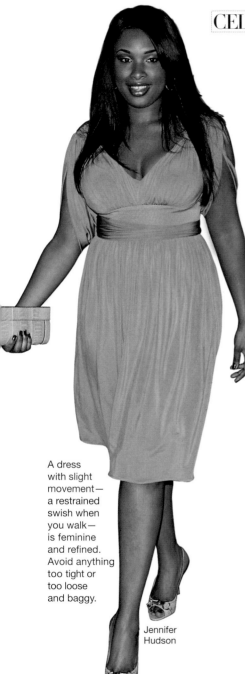

A dress with slight movement— a restrained swish when you walk— is feminine and refined. Avoid anything too tight or too loose and baggy.

Jennifer Hudson

- **Choose close-to-the-body cuts.** Caftans and sack or boxy shapes will only add pounds. Look for tailored pieces like fitted button-ups, straight skirts and trousers, and wrap dresses that skim the body and give the waist definition.
- **Keep it streamlined.** Your clothes should be sleek—frill free and not overly adorned. Think flat-front skirts and pants, as heavy pleats and too much volume look extra bulky. Pick tops that are relatively simple, without layers of ruffles and embellishment.
- **Don draping shapes.** While a structured look always works, pliable fabrics like jersey can be your best friend. You can wrap, twist, and gather a soft, stretchy fabric around your body so it highlights some parts and hides others.
- **Pick a basic palette.** Solid hues in lights or darks will serve you well. But don't avoid brights altogether. A rich red is always striking; ditto lush jewel tones. Big prints aren't best, so go monochromatic to create the slimmest line, or wear simple, contrasting shades like black and white.

"Accentuate your best features and disguise what you are not so happy with. Choose outfits that fit and make you look comfortable rather than those that are up-to-the-minute." —GIORGIO ARMANI

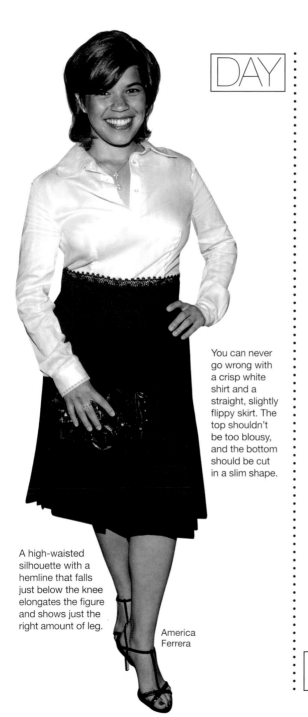

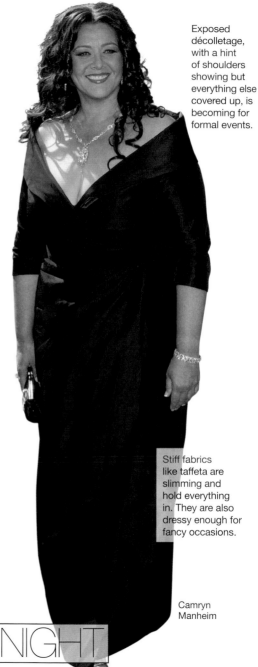

Exposed décolletage, with a hint of shoulders showing but everything else covered up, is becoming for formal events.

You can never go wrong with a crisp white shirt and a straight, slightly flippy skirt. The top shouldn't be too blousy, and the bottom should be cut in a slim shape.

Stiff fabrics like taffeta are slimming and hold everything in. They are also dressy enough for fancy occasions.

A high-waisted silhouette with a hemline that falls just below the knee elongates the figure and shows just the right amount of leg.

America Ferrera

Camryn Manheim

NIGHT

85

Boyish

The key is to create womanly curves and definition

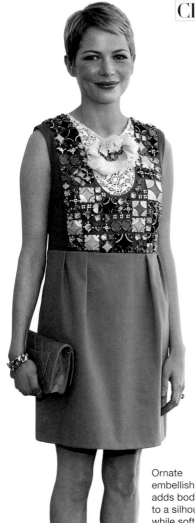

Ornate embellishment adds body to a silhouette, while soft pleats at the waist add a bit of fullness.

Michelle Williams

- **Enhance your figure.** To transform your slender physique into a more curvy shape, accentuate your middle and create the illusion of a fuller bust and hips. That means always define the waist, whether it's with a dress that cinches, a top with a drop waist, or a gown with a distinct Empire line. V-necks emphasize cleavage.
- **Turn up the volume.** Pieces with pleats, poufs, and peplums add ladylike definition. The same goes for anything with adornment. Ruffles, beading, and bows all offer a feminine boost to your figure. Balance anything with a lot of personality or dimension by pairing it with something more streamlined.
- **Play with prints.** Don't shy away from bold and intricate patterns. Florals, stripes, and graphics will give depth and character to a silhouette, but remember to keep it in check. Choose refined motifs in classic colors to keep from going overboard.
- **Trick the eye with details.** Accents like wide belts, ruching, and plays on color will give a touch more roundness to your shape. The same goes for a mix of textures: A combination of fabrics like lace, satin, velvet, cotton, and wool adds complexity to any silhouette.

> "If you select an outfit that you feel good wearing, then that's what people will notice." —DONATELLA VERSACE

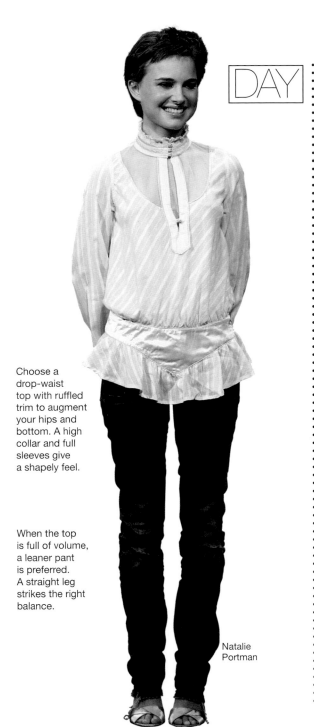

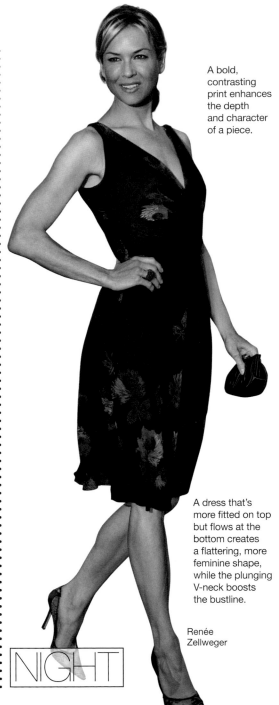

A bold, contrasting print enhances the depth and character of a piece.

Choose a drop-waist top with ruffled trim to augment your hips and bottom. A high collar and full sleeves give a shapely feel.

When the top is full of volume, a leaner pant is preferred. A straight leg strikes the right balance.

Natalie Portman

A dress that's more fitted on top but flows at the bottom creates a flattering, more feminine shape, while the plunging V-neck boosts the bustline.

Renée Zellweger

Petite

Work to elongate and enhance a small frame

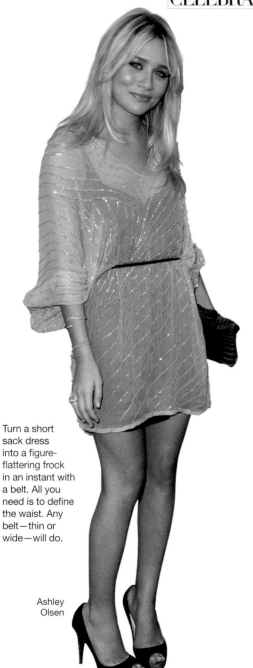

Turn a short sack dress into a figure-flattering frock in an instant with a belt. All you need is to define the waist. Any belt—thin or wide—will do.

Ashley Olsen

- **Heed hemlines.** A leggy look is sure to give you the appearance of a long, lean figure. Keep your short hemline in perspective: A mini a few inches above the knee may work for the younger crowd, while just above the knee is short enough for others. On the other hand, a longer skirt or dress that falls midcalf or even to the floor can elongate the silhouette if a high waist—that is, over the hips—is defined.
- **Keep the waist in focus.** Again, highlighting the middle is so important—especially for someone on the smaller side. Note that your true waistline, if not higher, should be the target point. A drop waist will only make you look shorter.
- **Stay solid.** Keep your look sleek and chic, and avoid very busy prints. You don't want to get lost in a loud pattern. Mixing solids works, and subtle details can add personality, but stay away from things, like overly ornate embellishment, that will detract from your figure.
- **Try lots of texture.** Plush fabrics like brocade, velvet, silk, lace, and chiffon can add character and fullness in the right places, and combining different fabrics will increase the richness of your look. Shun lots of layers, however, because your petite figure will look too loaded down. When in doubt, add three-inch heels!

> "Highlight the positive and delete the negative." —DONNA KARAN

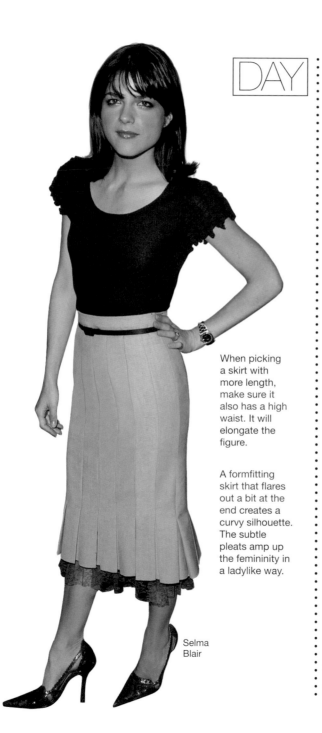

A ruffle trim on a strapless frock creates the look of a bigger bust, especially when offset by a supercinched waist. The wide sash enhances the hourglass.

When picking a skirt with more length, make sure it also has a high waist. It will elongate the figure.

A formfitting skirt that flares out a bit at the end creates a curvy silhouette. The subtle pleats amp up the femininity in a ladylike way.

Black opaque tights and equally dark shoes tone down the glitz factor of a metallic fabric and give the legs a longer look.

Selma Blair

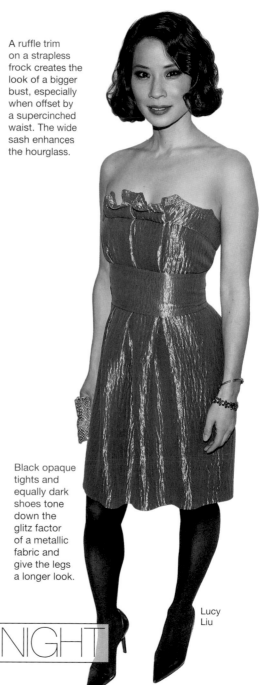

Lucy Liu

NIGHT

Pregnant

Keeping chic when you're expecting should be a cinch

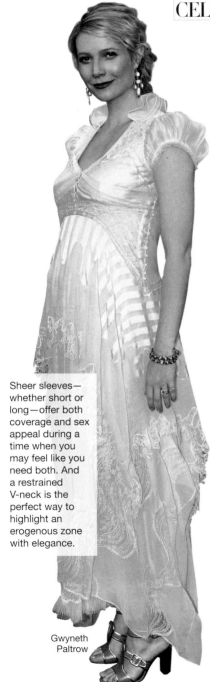

Sheer sleeves—whether short or long—offer both coverage and sex appeal during a time when you may feel like you need both. And a restrained V-neck is the perfect way to highlight an erogenous zone with elegance.

Gwyneth Paltrow

- **An Empire waist is a winner.** Just because your natural waistline has given way to a baby bump doesn't mean you should lose all definition. Cinch in the area just under the bust for the most flattering silhouette in tops, dresses, and even gowns. Maternity muumuus and tent dresses are a thing of the past.
- **Keep the cleavage in check.** By the time you are fully showing, no doubt your breasts will be larger than you are used to. Completely covering up will add pounds, while revealing too much will look sloppy. Find a happy medium with scoop necks, thick-strap tank cuts, and even V-necks with a little more coverage.
- **Find easy, breezy pieces.** Dresses, skirts, and tops that have swing are best for those with a baby on board. While tight tees and tanks may be a cute way to show off the belly, allow bottoms to have a little room and some movement. Make sure your tops fall at least to the hip so they cover the elastic waistband of your pants.
- **Keep it classic.** Crazy colors, prints, and embellishment look too over-the-top when you have a pregnant belly to contend with. Solids in simple light or dark hues are most polished.

> "If you are 20 pounds heavier than you normally are, go for women designers, because they cut clothes that are forgiving."
> —GWYNETH PALTROW

90

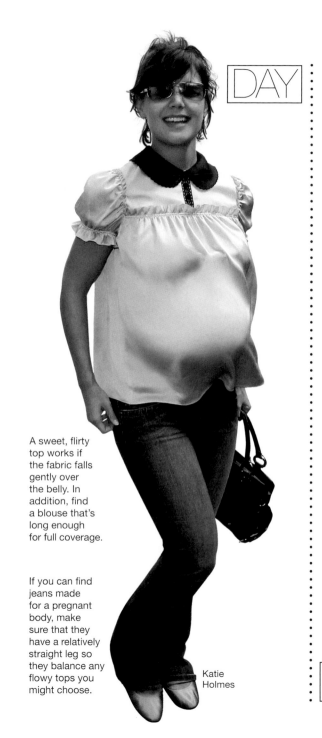

A sweet, flirty top works if the fabric falls gently over the belly. In addition, find a blouse that's long enough for full coverage.

If you can find jeans made for a pregnant body, make sure that they have a relatively straight leg so they balance any flowy tops you might choose.

Katie Holmes

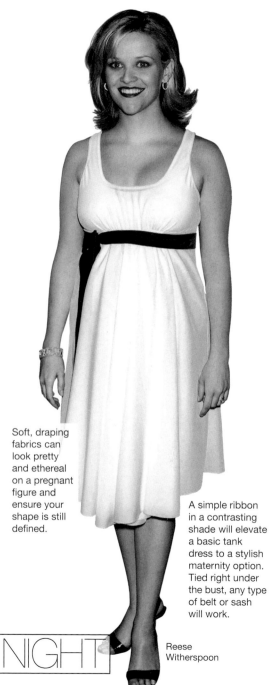

Soft, draping fabrics can look pretty and ethereal on a pregnant figure and ensure your shape is still defined.

A simple ribbon in a contrasting shade will elevate a basic tank dress to a stylish maternity option. Tied right under the bust, any type of belt or sash will work.

NIGHT

Reese Witherspoon

Accentuate Your Assets

Dressing well is not just about wearing the right clothes. It's about wearing the clothes that are right for your figure.

Have you ever noticed that some women never make a fashion misstep and always seem to be flawlessly pulled together? Take a closer look and you may notice that those whose sartorial sense you admire may wear the same style over and over. They know how to emphasize their assets, obscure what they aren't so proud of, and make their body look its absolute finest. Whether they're cinching in the waist on a jacket (to look more shapely), finding the perfect ratio of heel height to hemline length (to seem taller), or showing cleavage while covering up everywhere else (to draw attention away from the hips), some women know how to work their wardrobe to their advantage. Learn the tricks from those who've mastered the art of dressing the best for their body and make your clothes the most flattering they can be.

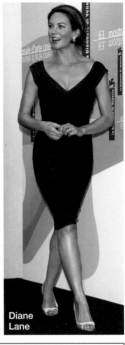

Diane Lane

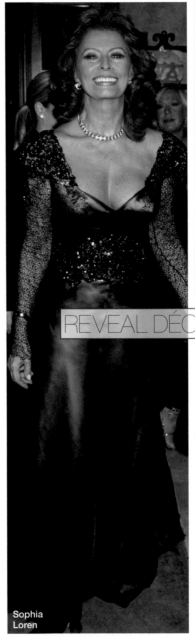

Sophia Loren

REVEAL DÉCOLLETAGE

- **Select a top that frames your neckline.** It will draw attention to your upper body, keeping the rest understated.

- **A formfitting black dress** with a strapless, off-the-shoulder, or wide-neck top is a dramatic look.

- **Wearing longer pieces** balances the intensity of an exposed top, maintaining proper proportions.

- **For a more casual take,** try low-cut blouses, wide-neck tanks, or tees paired with slim pants.

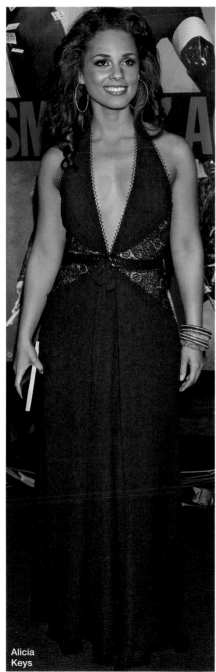

Alicia Keys

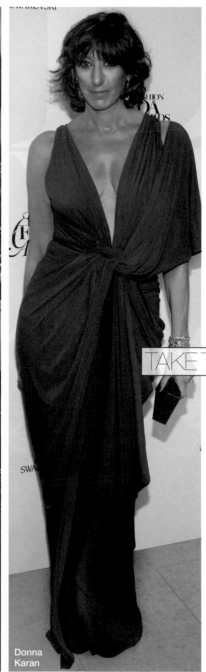

Donna Karan

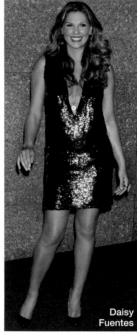

Daisy Fuentes

TAKE THE PLUNGE

- **A deep V on a gown,** a less severe dip on a cocktail dress, or even a slight plunge on a more casual top for day instantly detracts from your hips.

- **Make sure your bust is adequately secured in** and that a neckline provides enough coverage. Showing too much isn't sexy.

- **Keep your appearance appropriate** and in proportion by wearing more conservative bottoms, like trousers or a straight skirt. A dress should be simple with a drape.

- **Solid colors keep the look sleek** while allowing your cleavage to take center stage.

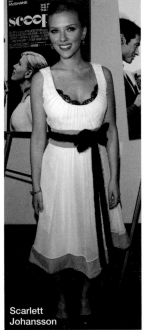

Scarlett
Johansson

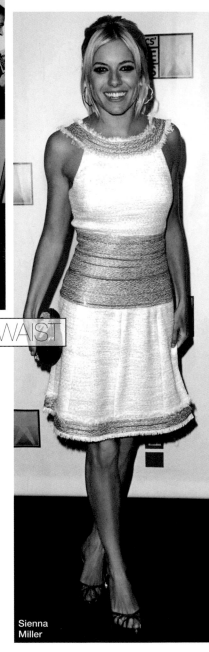

Sienna
Miller

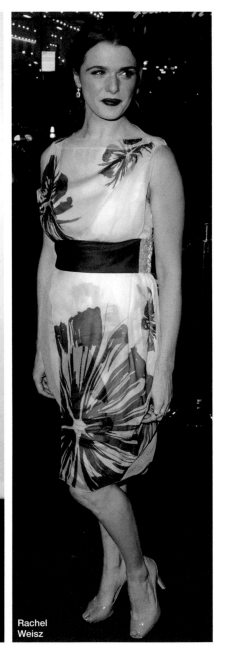

Rachel
Weisz

DEFINE THE WAIST

- **Whether you are tall or short,** a size 2 or a 12, cinching your middle almost always creates a feminine and flattering line.

- **Pick pieces with a slim belt or ribbon** for subtle definition. Or for a more dramatic effect, choose a superwide waistband like a cummerbund or obi-style sash.

- **The waist doesn't have to be smack in the middle.** A drop waist elongates your torso, while an Empire gives you a leggier look.

- **Details on the waist, like big bows,** work well in detracting the eye from your top or bottom.

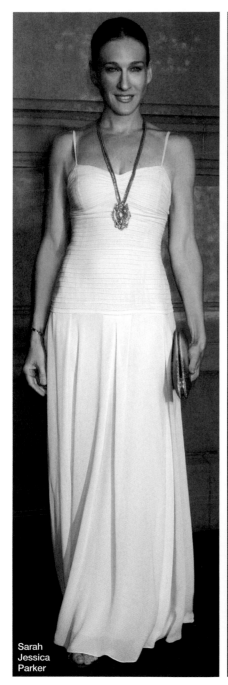

Sarah
Jessica
Parker

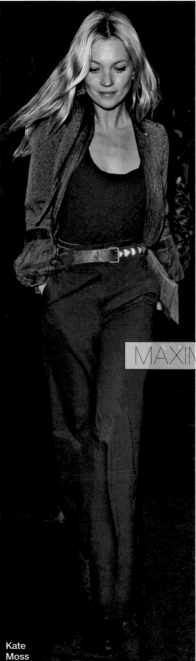

Kate
Moss

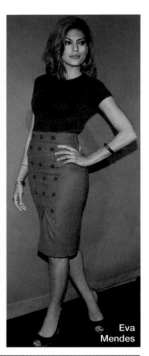

Eva
Mendes

MAXIMIZE HEIGHT

- **Floor-skimming frocks and trousers** will give you an elongated, lean look. Anything cropped at the ankle will shorten your silhouette.

- **Extremely high-waisted styles** will make your legs seem miles long. It's a good option when you prefer a midlength skirt.

- **Dressing in a single shade** optimizes your length. Strategic color-blocking can work well, too.

- **Avoid anything overly adorned or patterned.** The simpler the better when it comes to a streamlined look.

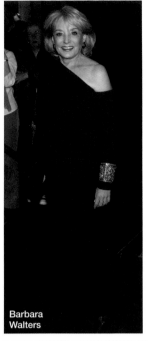

Barbara
Walters

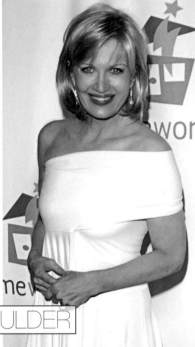

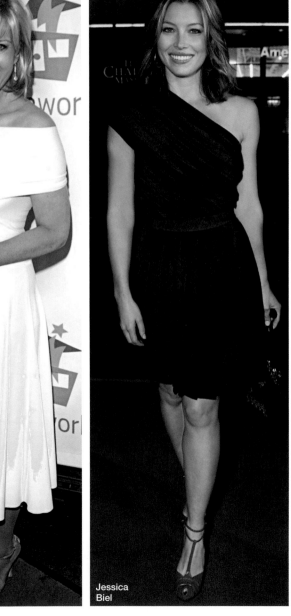

SHOW A SHOULDER

- **Reveal just one body part**—the back, a shoulder, or an arm—and keep the rest of yourself covered if you like to dress modestly without forsaking sex appeal.

- **Choose your most flattering asset** and dress to highlight it. Shoulders usually look lean and toned, even if the rest of you is not!

- **Halter dresses and asymmetrical styles** are ideal for showing just a little. Pick pieces in draping jersey that shield but simultaneously emphasize curves.

- **The effect works best in solids.** Loud colors, prints, and embellishments detract from the dramatic impact.

Diane
Sawyer

Jessica
Biel

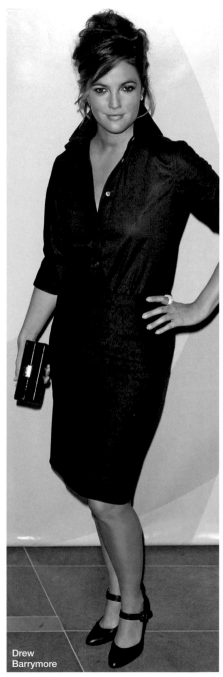

Drew
Barrymore

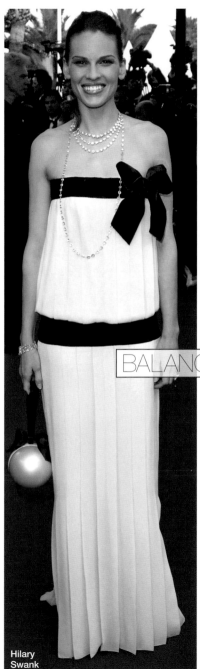

Hilary
Swank

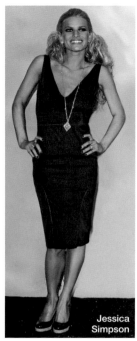

Jessica
Simpson

BALANCE THE BUST

- **Create a leaner look** by wearing an outfit in a solid dark shade.

- **Try tailored pieces like a classic button-up.** The structure of the shirt keeps everything looking sleek.

- **A moderate V-neck is a great shape** if you have a larger bust. It's a sultry way to show skin but keep the look modest. Anything too low could be inappropriate.

- **Strapless styles that lie flat can downplay a bigger bust.** One bold adornment, like a big bow or necklace, also helps— but loads of frills will just add bulk.

Universally Flattering Pieces

Some items of clothing look great on all shapes and sizes

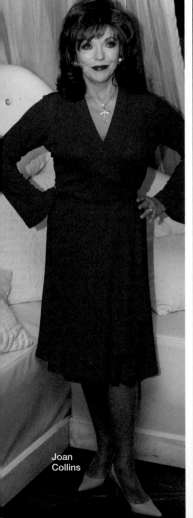

Joan Collins

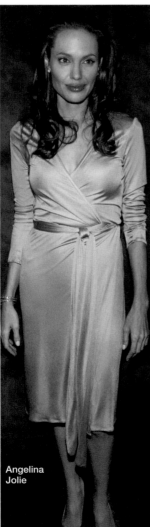

Angelina Jolie

WRAP DRESS

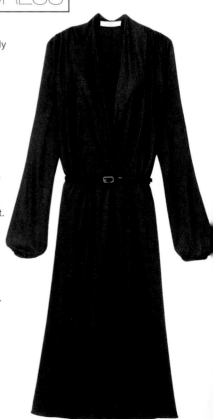

- **Soft jersey fabrics** can work for all body types. Twist, wrap, and maneuver the material any way you like to mask your least favorite parts and highlight the areas you like.

- **A woman with a very thin figure** can benefit from the draping fabric and the dress's ability to emphasize the waist.

- **A fuller-figured woman** looks great in the hour-glass-enhancing silhouette and the loosely falling fabric.

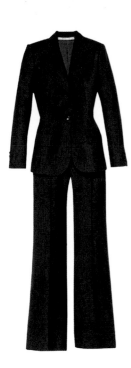

BLACK SUIT

- **First of all, it's black,** the ever-appealing, hide-everything hue. You can't go wrong.

- **Second, it's sturdy.** A well-cut, properly fitted jacket retains its shape, doesn't stretch or squeeze, and covers common problem areas like arms, stomach, hips, and bottom.

- **Last, depending on what you wear underneath,** the suit jacket can display just the right amount of skin around the neck and décolletage.

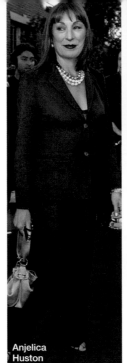

Anjelica Huston

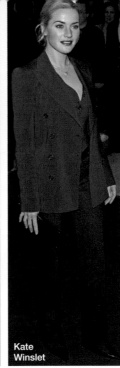

Kate Winslet

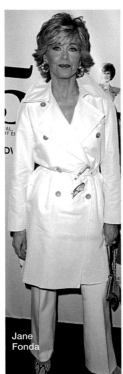

Jane Fonda

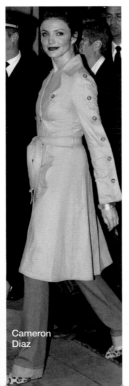

Cameron Diaz

TRENCH COAT

- **The tailored structure of this classic** hides all flaws, as does the stiff fabric.

- **The belt can be tied tight** to dramatically define the waist or loosely for a more casual air.

- **And the best part is,** the coat goes with everything—from jeans and a tee to a formal gown—and always looks chic.

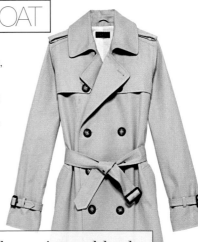

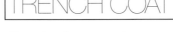

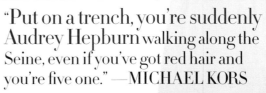

"Put on a trench, you're suddenly Audrey Hepburn walking along the Seine, even if you've got red hair and you're five one." —MICHAEL KORS

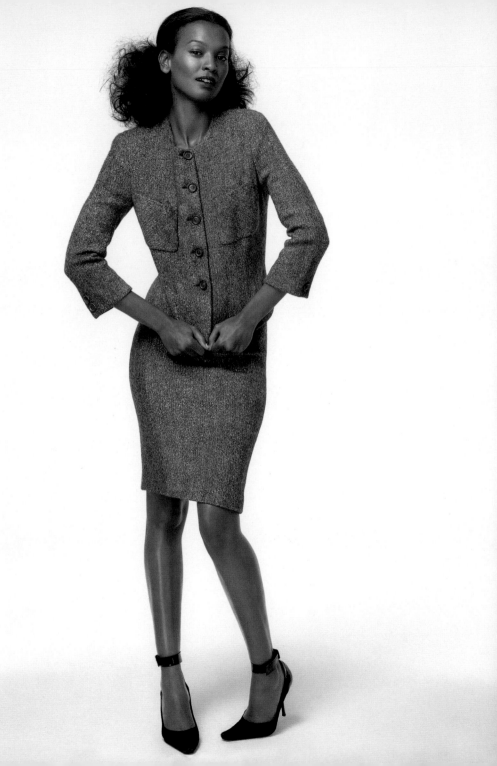

Office Elegance

5. Be confident in what you wear to work

"The difference between style and fashion is quality."

—GIORGIO ARMANI

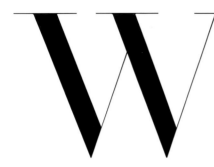

Whether you spend your day in front of a computer, in meetings, or at luncheons, dressing professionally and appropriately counts. These days, looking chic and tailored is not only about putting on the traditional two-piece suit, grabbing your structured bag, and slipping on those pointy pumps. Thankfully, fashion has become more interesting, and there are loads of exciting options out there that will pass muster even in a conservative office environment. So while many of us are restricted by our office dress code, that doesn't have to mean boring and basic.

The suit, for example, has come a long way from power shoulders and pleated matching bottoms. In fact, it can mean a lot of things to women of different ages. It can mean Kate Moss–esque skinny jeans with a tank and boyfriend blazer or superslim pants and a puff-sleeve blouse under a vest. Maybe a cropped jacket with a hint of swing and a tee casually peeking out worn with a pencil skirt is considered a suit to some, while it's full-leg trousers with a long, belted cardie for others. Then some women might prefer the more traditional two- or three-piece silhouette. Dresses should be factored in, too. They are an easy one-step option. The bottom line: Looking polished and pulled together is of the utmost importance when it comes to workwear.

Essential Supplies

What every working girl should have in her closet

Start with the right wardrobe foundation and getting dressed for work will be effortless. You can't go wrong with a stock of always-appropriate staples. Suits are a given, and with the right separates, you'll be all set. Keep in mind that black is a no-brainer, and you'll be fine if you stick with the standards in that shade. Otherwise, introduce gray, camel, and navy. Add tweedy styles for more variety.

1. Trousers
2. Blazers
3. Pencil skirts
4. White button-ups
5. Silk blouses
6. Simple cardigans
7. Dresses: shirt, shift, or sheath
8. Pumps
9. Structured bag
10. Belts

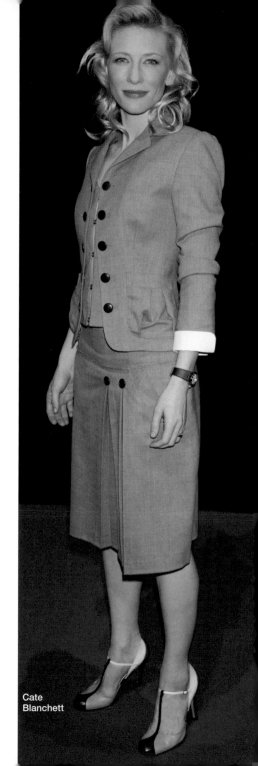

Cate Blanchett

Dress Code

Whether your place of work is strict or relaxed, there is a certain level of refinement that should always be maintained—and there are things you should simply never do

1. Obey the rules, whether you like them or not. Dressing against office dictates won't impress the boss—or your colleagues.

2. Never show your midriff. Wear shirts of a proper length, and shun pants that ride too low.

3. Avoid revealing too much cleavage. Work is definitely not the place for it.

4. Keep your straps under wraps. Never let your bra show, and make sure your shirt is buttoned up properly.

5. And don't wear anything see-through without proper underpinnings, ever.

6. Keep your hemlines in check. Even if you have great gams, supershort skirts should be saved for evenings out or weekends. A few inches above the knee is the shortest you should go.

7. Save your flip-flops for the beach. And your sneakers for the gym. Wear a pair of simple flats for your commute instead.

8. Use your best judgment: Save slinkier styles, like lacy camisoles and strapless dresses, for the evening.

9. Try not to go too tight. The office isn't the right place to hug *every* curve.

10. Don't get too wacky. It's fine to express your personal style, but keep it refined. Crazy hats, over-the-top makeup, and raucous patterns or colors will make you seem too eccentric.

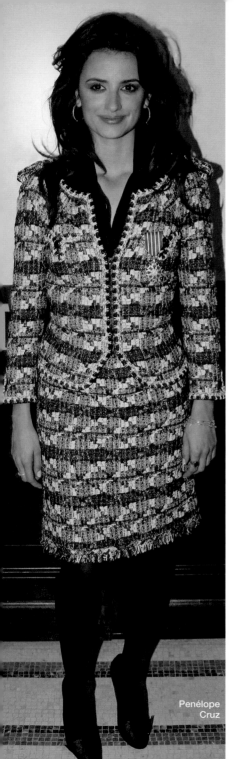

Penélope
Cruz

Suits
Timeless & Tailored

The traditional two-piece is the standard. In a well-cut jacket with matching pants or a skirt, you know you'll always look smart.

Whether you rely on one as your everyday answer to dressing or consider it a once-in-a-while option, a suit is a must-have. There is a reason it has never gone out of style. Yes, trends in suits have flowed from dramatic proportions, with big shoulders and slouchy cuts to superlean lines and back again, but a finely cut, precisely tailored suit, either basic or gussied up, assuredly looks good. The right one can give you confidence, a sense of power, and instant polish. It offers a never-fail solution when you are hit with a what-to-wear crisis. Most of all, it's dependable for work—always appropriate, easy to wear, and no-nonsense. Plus, there is a suit to flatter every one of us. Stick to the classics and you can't go wrong.

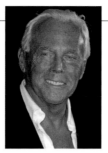

Giorgio Armani
On How to Wear a Suit

What tried-and-true fashion tips can you impart?
Do not mix too many strong features. A beautifully tailored suit is complete with one or two accessories, no more. A subtle look is more intriguing. Design does not need to be overcomplicated or dramatic to make a big impact.

What essentials should every woman own?
The suit should be the key element in any woman's wardrobe. A beautifully tailored jacket, a white shirt, and a pair of flowing trousers are the perfect items for any occasion. Also, a slimming pair of dark denim jeans can be both casual and chic if paired properly.

When do you know it's time to buy a new suit?
Modern women are looking for special individual pieces that are easily mixed with other things in their wardrobe. In this way, you can make up a new "suit" for any occasion without always buying a new one! Do, however, pay attention to wear and tear. The pants might last longer than the jacket, but a suit can also be split up or renewed by replacing one of the items.

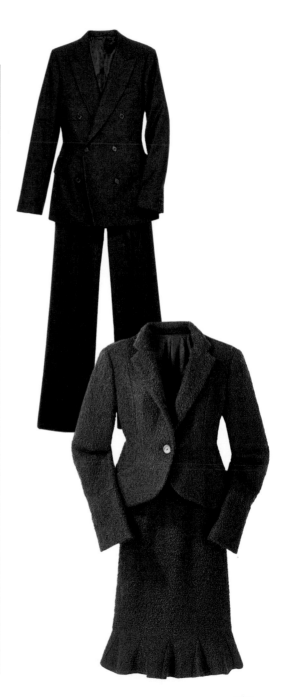

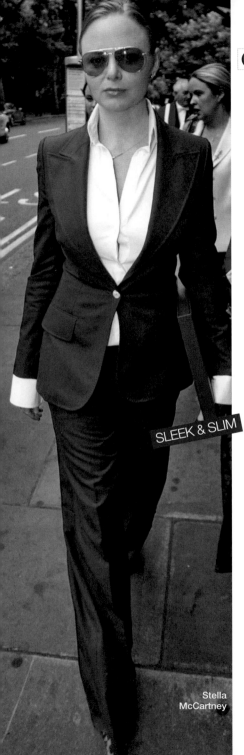

SLEEK & SLIM

Stella
McCartney

Pant-suits

These borrowed-from-the-boys, workworthy outfits should have a prominent place in your professional wardrobe

While the pantsuit is as classic as it gets, you'd be surprised how many forms this basic can take. There's the sleek silhouette that looks modern and severe; the wide-leg, slouchy style with a retro air; the banker look of pinstripes or checks; and the old-fashioned tweed that recalls the English countryside, to name a few. Meanwhile, a simple, no-frills suit can be a blank canvas for creating any style you want. The important thing is to choose the look that you feel comfortable in and is most appropriate for your place of work. No matter which pantsuit is best for you, always balance the masculine cut with a feminine touch, whether it's a ruffled blouse, a hint of lace, or a well-defined waist.

"Simplicity always shows off the woman."
—MICHAEL KORS

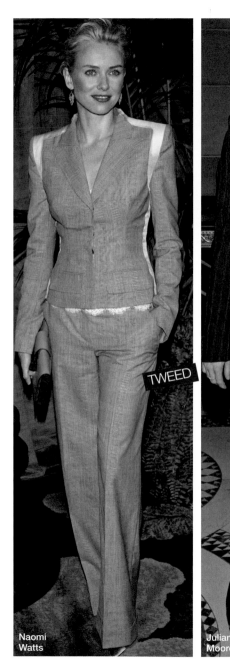

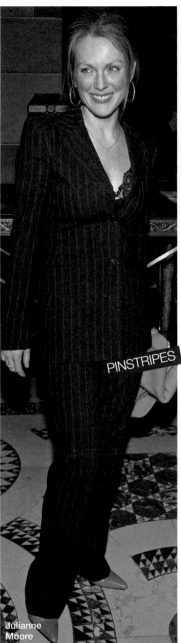

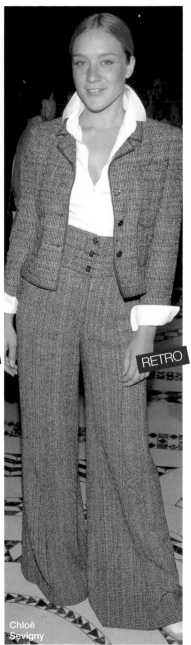

TWEED

PINSTRIPES

RETRO

Naomi
Watts

Julianne
Moore

Chloë
Sevigny

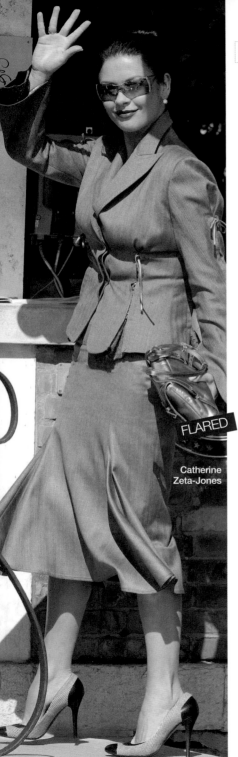

FLARED

Catherine
Zeta-Jones

Skirt Suits

Choose the ever-chic basic with a feminine spin

Just because you're wearing a suit doesn't mean you have to sacrifice your sex appeal. A matching skirt and jacket provide the perfect balance between looking serious and womanly. They also come in an endless variety of styles. A prim bouclé suit says ladylike, a sleek, body-hugging cut can look sultry, and a boxy shape in a nubby tweed has a retro feel. When searching for the best silhouette for you, start with the line of the skirt—from a slim pencil to a pleated dirndl—and work around it. It's important that the jacket balances well with the shape of the skirt. A fuller skirt, for example, looks best with a fitted jacket. If you prefer a jacket that makes more of a statement and has, say, a flared peplum, choose a body-conscious skirt to go with it. The hemline should also be considered. You can't go wrong with to-the-knee or an inch above or below. Ankle-length skirts are rarely flattering in terms of suits, and minis are never appropriate for the office.

> "Dress smart and feminine. There are certain things that don't look right in an office—miniskirts, décolletage, nakedness."
> —CAROLINA HERRERA

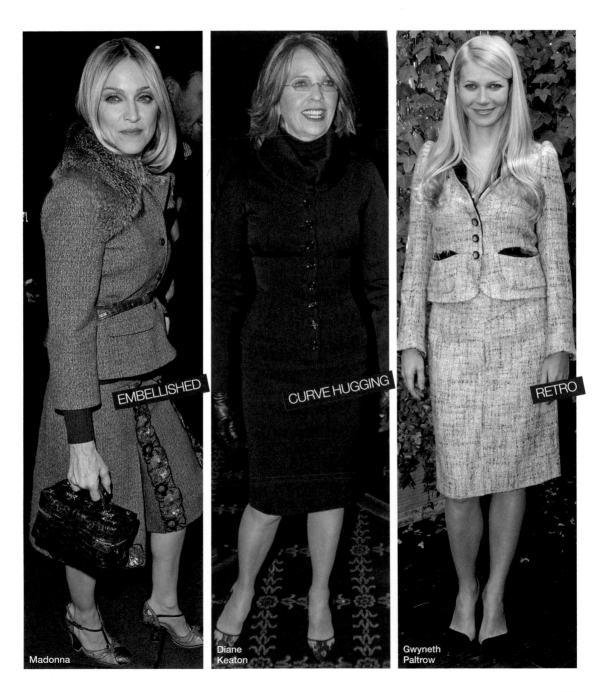

EMBELLISHED

CURVE HUGGING

RETRO

Madonna

Diane
Keaton

Gwyneth
Paltrow

111

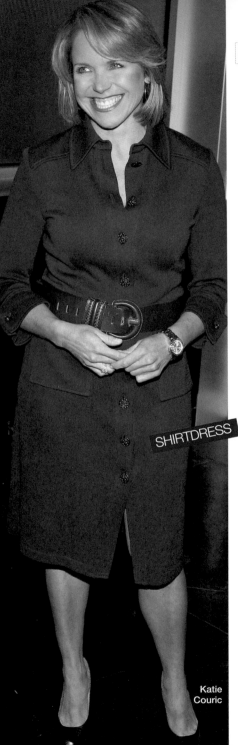

Katie
Couric

SHIRTDRESS

Workworthy Dresses

A clean-cut frock can look smart, sophisticated, and serious yet couldn't be simpler to wear

When it comes to dressing professionally, polish is what it's all about. And that isn't restricted to suits. The right dress can say power just as much as a suit, and since frocks are an all-in-one outfit, they are even easier to wear than a suit. There is no need to save them for nights out or weekends. The best dresses for work are refined and reserved. Think simple shifts, structured shirtdresses, and belted sheaths. You don't want to wear anything too tight, showy, or flashy. Neutral and dark hues—black, navy, browns—in solids are best, as are classic silhouettes. While dresses in general are perfect for women of all ages, use your common sense when picking what's right for you and what meets office guidelines. Younger women can often get away with slightly higher hemlines and bared shoulders, while those a bit older may want to choose more conservative cuts. Top off your frock with a cardigan, basic blazer, or matching coat that ends at the hem of your dress, not above.

> "It's the ease of one-piece dressing. Just put it on and you're done. A dress is less complicated and can be very chic."
> —FRANCISCO COSTA

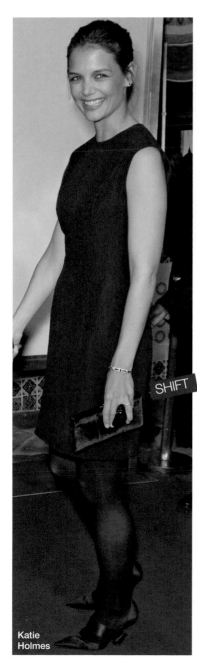

SHIFT

Katie
Holmes

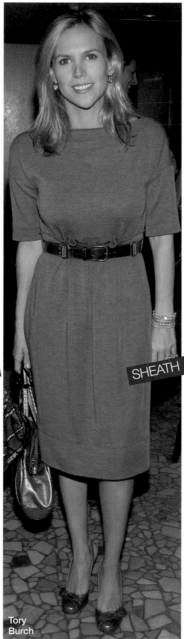

SHEATH

Tory
Burch

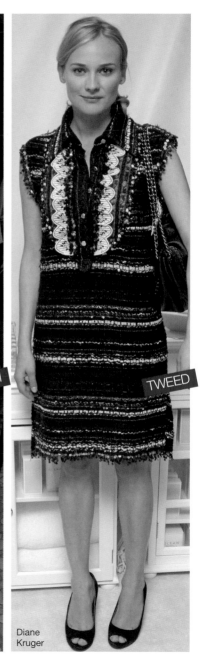

TWEED

Diane
Kruger

The Perfect Suit for Your Shape

There is a flattering fit for everyone. Find what works best for your body type.

The traditional jacket-and-skirt pairing can be a very becoming outfit. The tailored topper can discreetly hide your arms, your belly, and even your bottom, while a pencil skirt can accentuate curves and an A-line can mask them. But every cut is different, and it's important to pay attention to those nuances when finding the right fit for you.

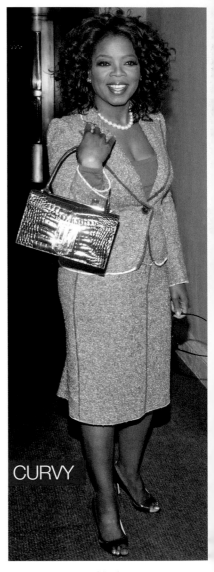

CURVY

A straight skirt and jacket provide a flattering fit. Avoid full or pleated skirts, as they'll just add bulk. The same goes for jackets: A well-cut piece that is close to the body (but not too tight) is much more complementary than a boxy, big-shouldered style.

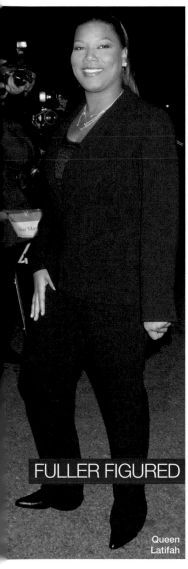

FULLER FIGURED

Queen
Latifah

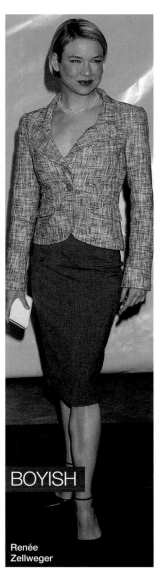

BOYISH

Renée
Zellweger

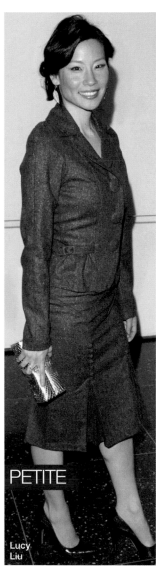

PETITE

Lucy
Liu

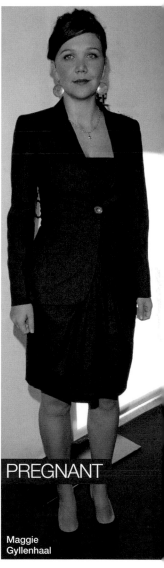

PREGNANT

Maggie
Gyllenhaal

A sleek, streamlined suit will never fail you. Your jacket should be tailored and trim and hit at the hips. Anything oversize won't look sharp. Straight-cut pants that fall to the bottom of your heel look best. Dark colors are flattering, but don't feel tied to them.

The important thing is to emphasize your waist and create curves, therefore a trim, slightly cropped jacket looks best. Pair it with a figure-enhancing skirt—one that tapers a touch and falls just below the knee. Try a two-toned suit or one with a textured fabric to add richness.

Stick to slim cuts. Anything big, boxy, or oversize will overwhelm your small physique. Stay away from big-shouldered, long jackets, and try pieces that are more fitted. Choose skirts that hit at the knee or an inch above or below—not longer. Dark solids will let your shape show.

Just because you have a bulging belly doesn't mean you can't have a streamlined silhouette. The key is finding the right jacket shape. A single-button blazer that closes just under the bust is flattering, while an A-line skirt might be most comfortable.

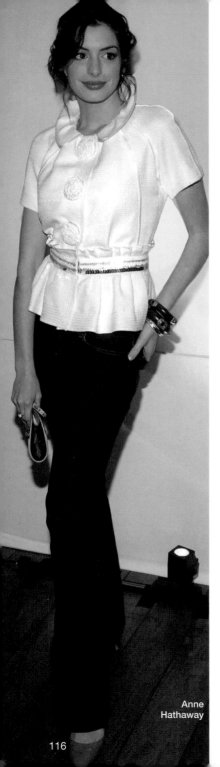

Fabulous at Every Age:
New Suits

When the dress code is less conservative, there are many polished alternatives to a traditional two-piece

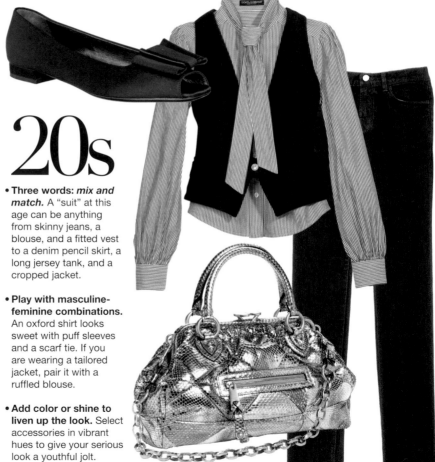

20s

- **Three words: *mix and match.*** A "suit" at this age can be anything from skinny jeans, a blouse, and a fitted vest to a denim pencil skirt, a long jersey tank, and a cropped jacket.

- **Play with masculine-feminine combinations.** An oxford shirt looks sweet with puff sleeves and a scarf tie. If you are wearing a tailored jacket, pair it with a ruffled blouse.

- **Add color or shine to liven up the look.** Select accessories in vibrant hues to give your serious look a youthful jolt.

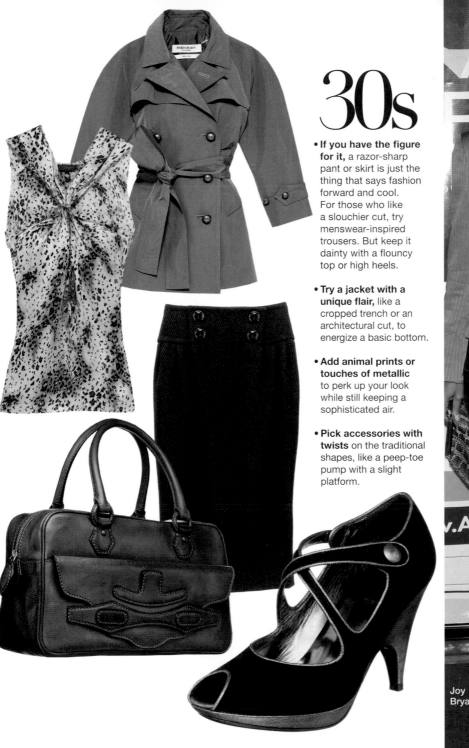

30s

- **If you have the figure for it,** a razor-sharp pant or skirt is just the thing that says fashion forward and cool. For those who like a slouchier cut, try menswear-inspired trousers. But keep it dainty with a flouncy top or high heels.

- **Try a jacket with a unique flair,** like a cropped trench or an architectural cut, to energize a basic bottom.

- **Add animal prints or touches of metallic** to perk up your look while still keeping a sophisticated air.

- **Pick accessories with twists** on the traditional shapes, like a peep-toe pump with a slight platform.

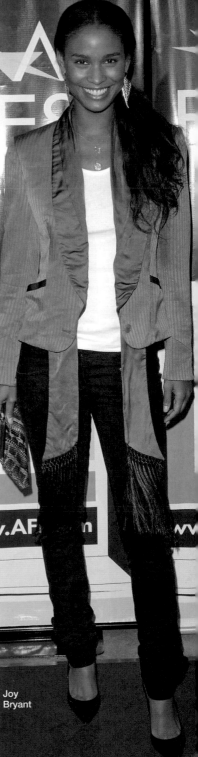

Joy Bryant

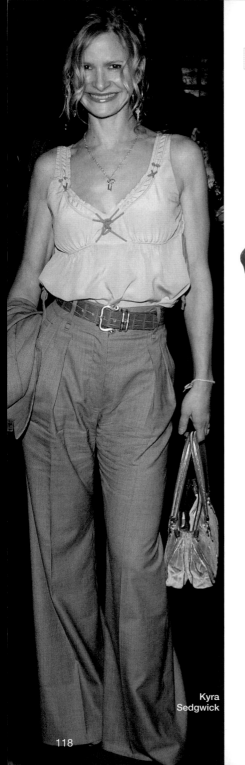

118

OFFICE ELEGANCE

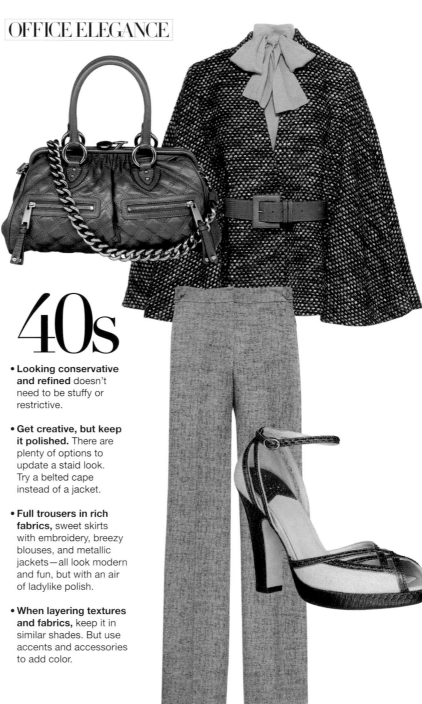

40s

- **Looking conservative and refined** doesn't need to be stuffy or restrictive.

- **Get creative, but keep it polished.** There are plenty of options to update a staid look. Try a belted cape instead of a jacket.

- **Full trousers in rich fabrics,** sweet skirts with embroidery, breezy blouses, and metallic jackets—all look modern and fun, but with an air of ladylike polish.

- **When layering textures and fabrics,** keep it in similar shades. But use accents and accessories to add color.

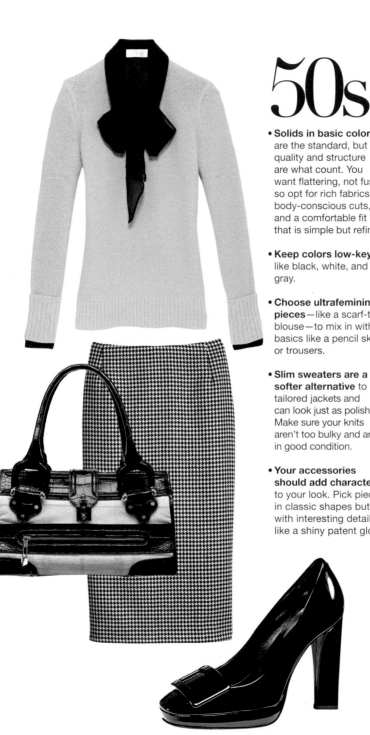

50s

- **Solids in basic colors** are the standard, but quality and structure are what count. You want flattering, not fussy, so opt for rich fabrics, body-conscious cuts, and a comfortable fit that is simple but refined.

- **Keep colors low-key,** like black, white, and gray.

- **Choose ultrafeminine pieces**—like a scarf-tied blouse—to mix in with basics like a pencil skirt or trousers.

- **Slim sweaters are a softer alternative** to tailored jackets and can look just as polished. Make sure your knits aren't too bulky and are in good condition.

- **Your accessories should add character** to your look. Pick pieces in classic shapes but with interesting details, like a shiny patent gloss.

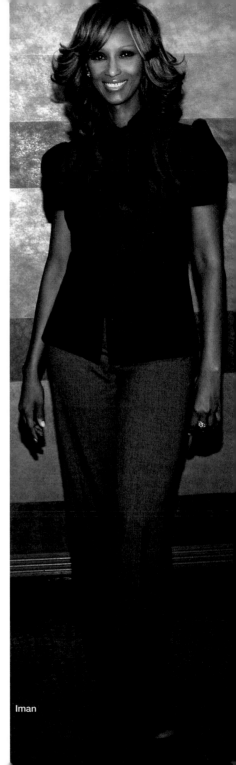

Iman

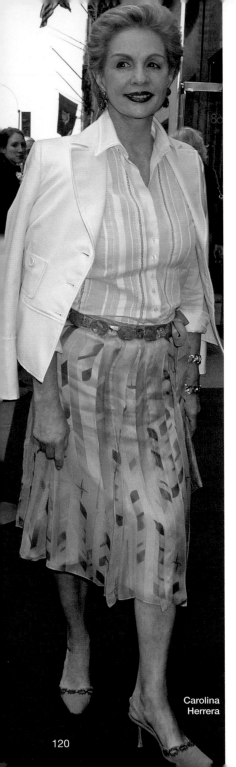

Carolina
Herrera

OFFICE ELEGANCE

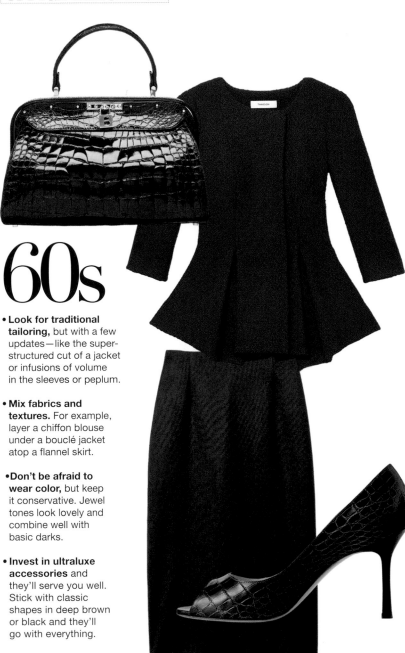

60s

- **Look for traditional tailoring,** but with a few updates—like the super-structured cut of a jacket or infusions of volume in the sleeves or peplum.

- **Mix fabrics and textures.** For example, layer a chiffon blouse under a bouclé jacket atop a flannel skirt.

- **Don't be afraid to wear color,** but keep it conservative. Jewel tones look lovely and combine well with basic darks.

- **Invest in ultraluxe accessories** and they'll serve you well. Stick with classic shapes in deep brown or black and they'll go with everything.

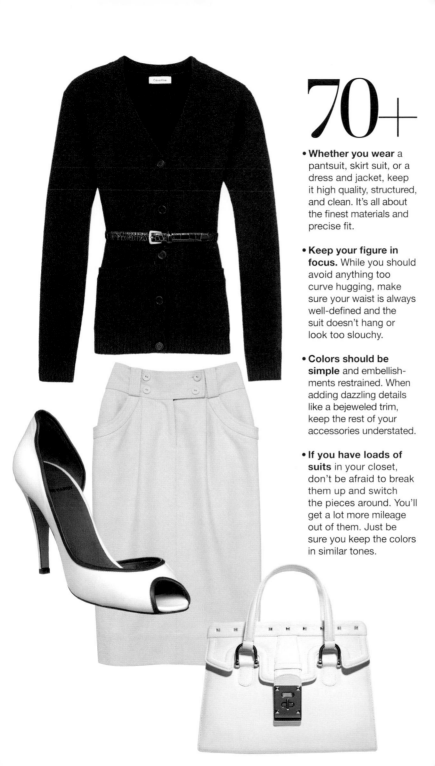

70+

- **Whether you wear** a pantsuit, skirt suit, or a dress and jacket, keep it high quality, structured, and clean. It's all about the finest materials and precise fit.

- **Keep your figure in focus.** While you should avoid anything too curve hugging, make sure your waist is always well-defined and the suit doesn't hang or look too slouchy.

- **Colors should be simple** and embellishments restrained. When adding dazzling details like a bejeweled trim, keep the rest of your accessories understated.

- **If you have loads of suits** in your closet, don't be afraid to break them up and switch the pieces around. You'll get a lot more mileage out of them. Just be sure you keep the colors in similar tones.

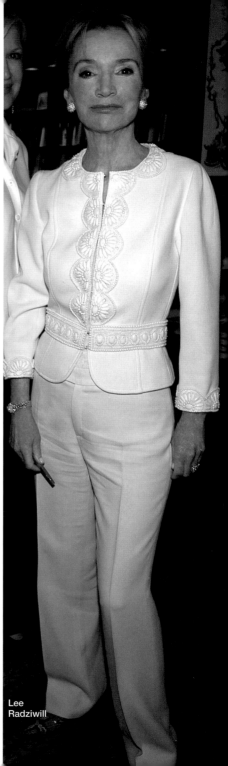

Lee Radziwill

Freshen Up Your Basics

Have an old suit hanging in your closet? Learn to perk it up and make it look new again with a few strategic updates.

While suits are an easy-to-wear fashion solution, they do have their drawbacks, hefty price tags being one of them. Tailoring and quality come at a price, so many of us can't afford many options. Also, those of us who have limited choice when it comes to suits are likely faced with another drawback: A suit can be boring. But don't fret if you have one go-to black suit in your closet. There are lots of ways to reinvent that old standby. Been wearing a basic button-up under your suit every day? Swap it for a bright blouse, something with loads of ruffles cascading down the front, or a piece with a bold print and it'll instantly add new life to that old suit.

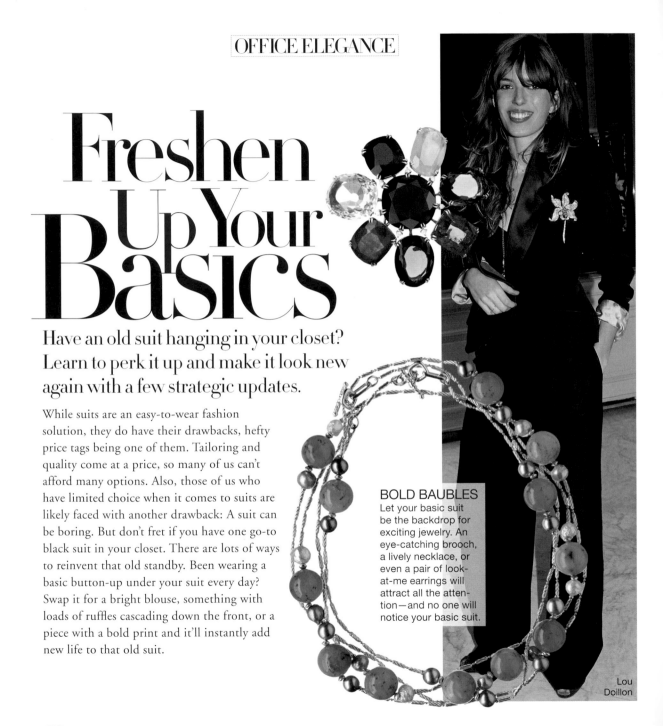

BOLD BAUBLES
Let your basic suit be the backdrop for exciting jewelry. An eye-catching brooch, a lively necklace, or even a pair of look-at-me earrings will attract all the attention—and no one will notice your basic suit.

Lou Doillon

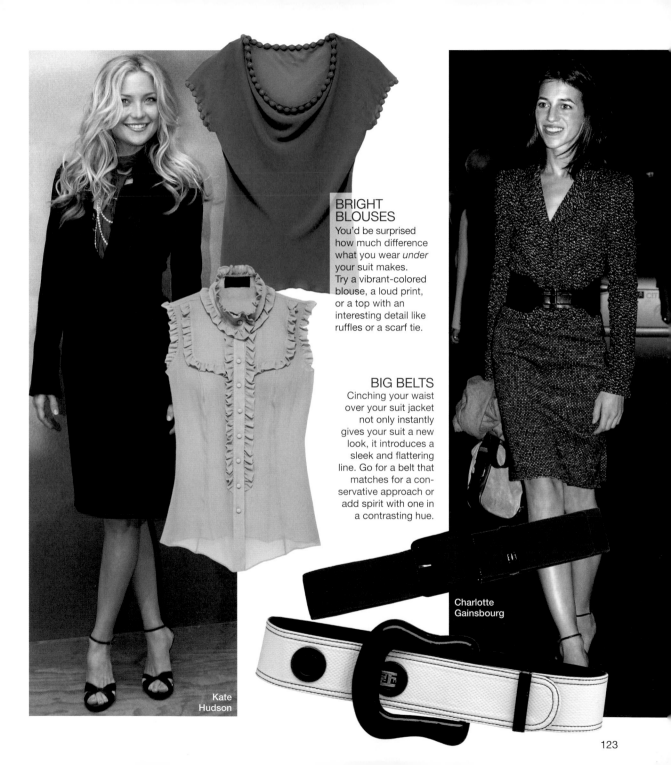

BRIGHT BLOUSES

You'd be surprised how much difference what you wear *under* your suit makes. Try a vibrant-colored blouse, a loud print, or a top with an interesting detail like ruffles or a scarf tie.

BIG BELTS

Cinching your waist over your suit jacket not only instantly gives your suit a new look, it introduces a sleek and flattering line. Go for a belt that matches for a conservative approach or add spirit with one in a contrasting hue.

Kate Hudson

Charlotte Gainsbourg

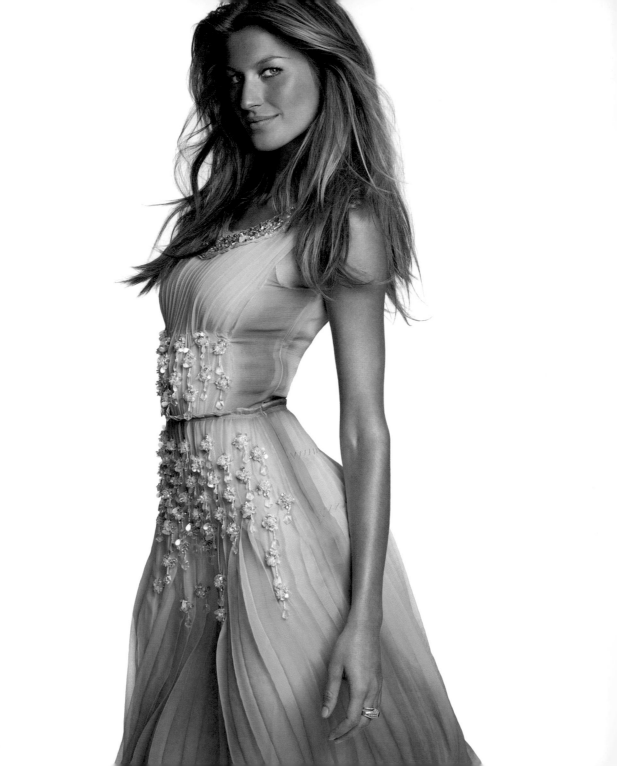

Evening Glam

6. Master a party-perfect look

"The only **real elegance** is in the **mind;** if you've got that, the rest really comes from it."
—DIANA VREELAND

There is nothing worse than arriving at a party and realizing you are wearing the wrong thing— that you will be tucking in your bra strap all night, that all eyes will be on your cleavage because your frock is plunging way too low, that the leopard print you picked doesn't actually say chic, it in fact screams, "Not me!" We've all been there before, unfortunately. So, what exactly makes for the perfect evening outfit? It's something you put on and don't have to think about again (until you're accepting compliments on it). It's an outfit you feel sexy in, not provocative; one you can wear with confidence without feeling like a peacock; one that lets you hit the dance floor with ease. It's never fussy or ill fitting. When you are dressed up for a party, you want to be yourself—or a better version of yourself. The perfect outfit allows your personality and beauty to shine through. How do you go about finding it? You must choose something that reflects your personal style and, of course, fits and flatters you.

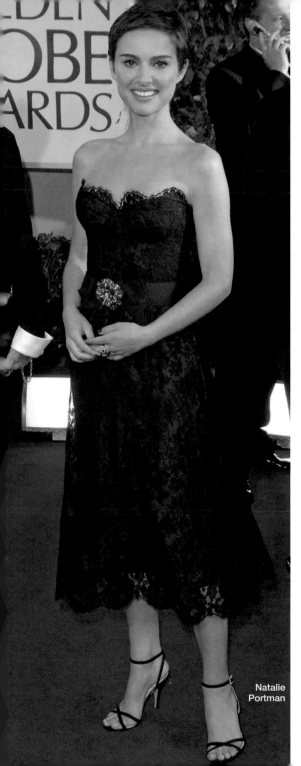

Natalie
Portman

Quick tips for a simply chic nighttime look:

- **Richness rules.** Choose pieces in lush textures like velvet, lace, and brocade for an instant special-occasion feel.

- **Go bright or shimmery.** A vibrant frock in a candy color is an immediate mood lifter, and anything metallic or sparkly will make you feel like a star.

- **Find something that's fuss free.** Avoid shoes you can't walk in, for example, and a dress that doesn't hold everything in.

- **Master the art of the office touch-up.** Wear just a little makeup that day so it looks fresh when you reapply before you go out. Spritz yourself with fragrance, too, for an extra boost.

- **When in doubt, stick with the basics.** You can't go wrong with that little black dress and a strappy sandal.

> "It shows confidence to wear a simple, graceful dress that is not calling attention to itself. Not showy, not flashy, just confidence that the woman herself will attract the gaze."
> —NATALIE PORTMAN

Going-Out Guidelines

When stepping out at night—whether for an intimate dinner or a posh cocktail party—always dress to keep your poise

1. **Consider comfort first and foremost.** Yes, you want to look a little sweet, sexy, and sophisticated—but if you are pained in what you are wearing, it'll show.

2. **Find an outfit that fits well.** Don't go too tight, or you'll look stuffed in your clothes, but don't go so loose that your figure gets lost.

3. **If you want to garner lots of attention,** go ahead and wear something that really stands out—but make sure it's polished and not over-the-top.

4. **If you want to be a wallflower,** pick something that's simple and understated, but it still should be chic.

5. **When wearing a basic, like your favorite LBD,** give it a personal touch—a funky brooch, a colorful scarf, a big necklace—to make it uniquely you.

6. Experimenting is encouraged—but road test a new look to make sure it works for you before you get to the party.

7. Respect the suggested dress code of the evening, but don't feel obligated to abide by it. Wear long to cocktails or short to a formal event—but style it in a way so you don't feel over- or underdressed.

8. Don't sweat it if you are in fact way off from the dress code. Be prepared for quick fixes. Too dressy for laid-back cocktails? Put your hair in a ponytail and toss a coat or a sweater over your shoulders. Or just say you have a more formal event to go to next!

9. Avoid anything fussy. It will bring you down. A long train that people could step on, feathers that make you sneeze, or a corset cut so you can't eat or breathe is certainly distracting—for you and others.

10. No matter what you wear, go with it and forget about it at the door. Being self-conscious and worrying about your look will detract from the fun you should be having.

Timeless Allure

Stunning after-sundown looks that have spanned the decades

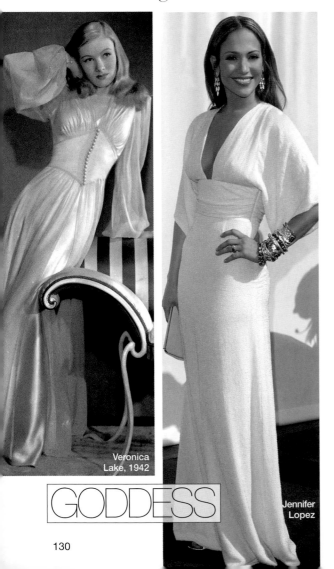

Veronica Lake, 1942

Jennifer Lopez

GODDESS

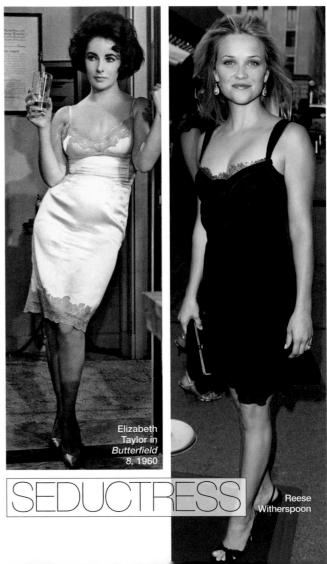

Elizabeth Taylor in *Butterfield 8*, 1960

Reese Witherspoon

SEDUCTRESS

Certain dresses—from flirty frocks to gorgeous gowns—have proven their ability to turn heads year after year. Choose one for your evening out and you are guaranteed to shine, just like red-carpet icons of the past and present.

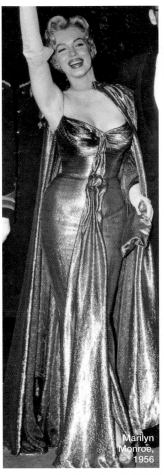

Marilyn Monroe, 1956

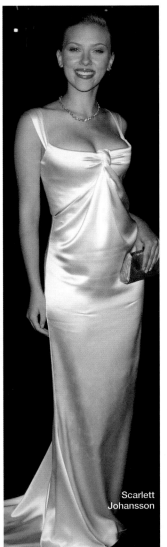

Scarlett Johansson

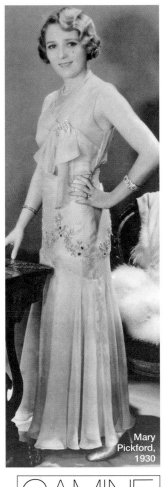

Mary Pickford, 1930

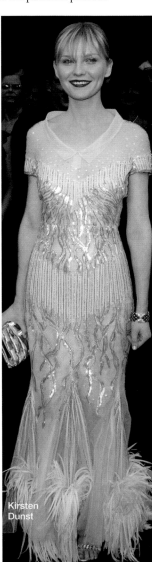

Kirsten Dunst

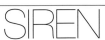

SIREN

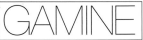

GAMINE

The Little Black Dress

It's the tried and true, the one you can forever rely on, the piece that never goes out of style

The little black dress has long been a standby, the item you pull out of your closet when you want to look instantly chic, classic, slim, sultry—or you just can't think of what else to wear. It's also a transformative must-have. There are endless styles and incarnations out there, from ornately jeweled numbers to slinky strappy cuts, to satisfy your every mood. Or you can take your favorite cut and dress it up or down to suit your latest whim. Think of your LBD as a blank canvas that you can decorate based on your age, frame of mind, or event. Shoes are the easiest way to update your dress. Jewelry is a definite mood setter as well. The choices are endless—whether you buy a new frock or give the one you have an of-the-moment makeover. Either way, you know you'll look great in that LBD.

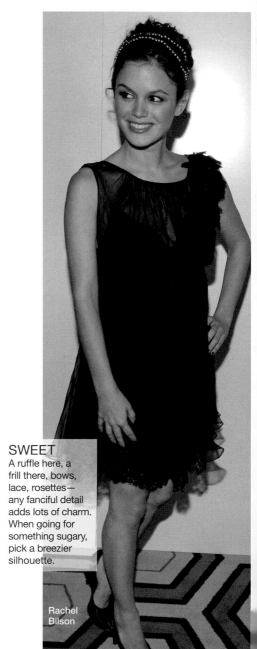

SWEET
A ruffle here, a frill there, bows, lace, rosettes—any fanciful detail adds lots of charm. When going for something sugary, pick a breezier silhouette.

Rachel Bilson

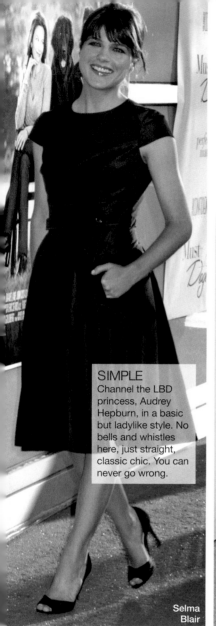

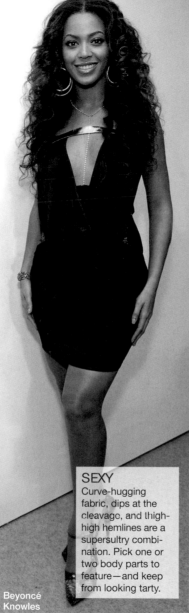

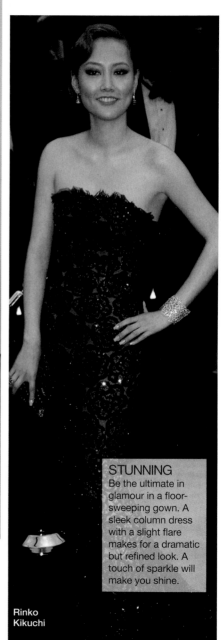

SIMPLE
Channel the LBD princess, Audrey Hepburn, in a basic but ladylike style. No bells and whistles here, just straight, classic chic. You can never go wrong.

Selma Blair

SEXY
Curve-hugging fabric, dips at the cleavage, and thigh-high hemlines are a supersultry combination. Pick one or two body parts to feature—and keep from looking tarty.

Beyoncé Knowles

STUNNING
Be the ultimate in glamour in a floor-sweeping gown. A sleek column dress with a slight flare makes for a dramatic but refined look. A touch of sparkle will make you shine.

Rinko Kikuchi

"The black dress is the embodiment of women's power. It's very stark, direct, and to the point." — ALEXANDER McQUEEN

GET THE LOOK

The Little Black Dress

FLIRTY
A mini is a fun and sexy LBD option. But with high hemlines, a simple cut on top, like a tank, keeps it from looking too provocative.

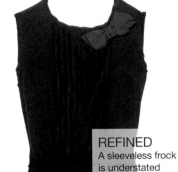

DAY-TO-NIGHT
A short-sleeved dress is charming *and* versatile. Layer a tank underneath for day if it's low cut.

REFINED
A sleeveless frock is understated and elegant. Pick something with a slight swing in the skirt for added femininity.

SLINKY
A slim, formfitting slipdress is all about subtle sultriness. A touch of beading adds to the flapper-era feel.

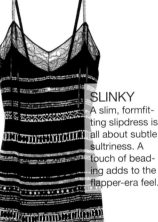

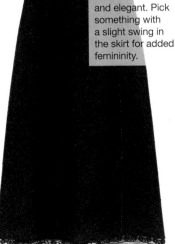

SWEETHEART
The '80s strapless style still looks good, but instead of a blown-up pouf, a leaner skirt looks more modern.

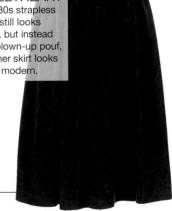

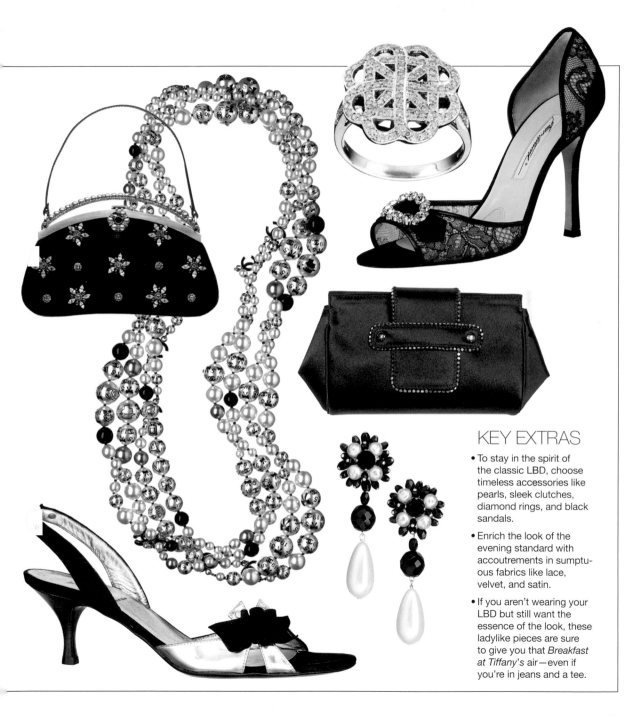

KEY EXTRAS

- To stay in the spirit of the classic LBD, choose timeless accessories like pearls, sleek clutches, diamond rings, and black sandals.

- Enrich the look of the evening standard with accoutrements in sumptuous fabrics like lace, velvet, and satin.

- If you aren't wearing your LBD but still want the essence of the look, these ladylike pieces are sure to give you that *Breakfast at Tiffany's* air—even if you're in jeans and a tee.

Night Brights

Black isn't the only option when it comes to dressing up. Stand out from the pack in a rainbow-hued frock.

When you are going out at night—for dinner, drinks, or dancing—the goal is to relax and have a good time. And we all know that what we wear has a big impact on how we feel. So, how to dress for a fun-filled evening? In cotton-candy pink, sunny yellow, marigold orange, electric blue, and lipstick red. Technicolor hues are instant mood lifters. Plus, when everyone else at the party is donned in dark shades, you'll be the one who stands out. When going for a bold hue, however, it doesn't have to be blindingly bright. Rich jewel tones like emerald, garnet, and sapphire are sophisticated and elegant. Remember, solids look best when going for big color in the evening.

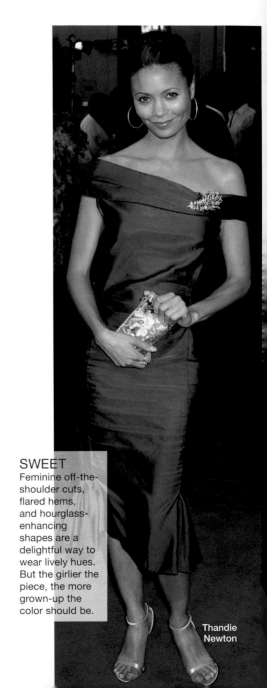

SWEET
Feminine off-the-shoulder cuts, flared hems, and hourglass-enhancing shapes are a delightful way to wear lively hues. But the girlier the piece, the more grown-up the color should be.

Thandie Newton

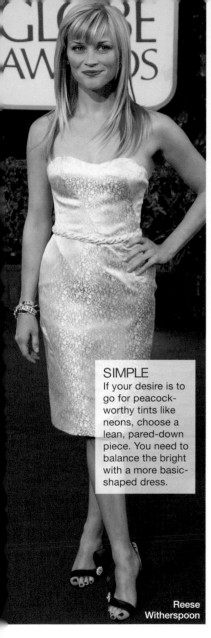

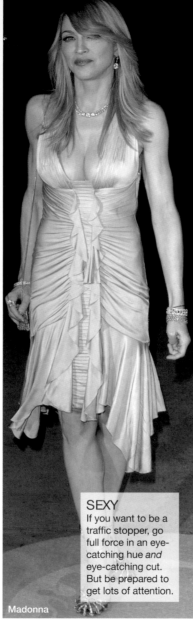

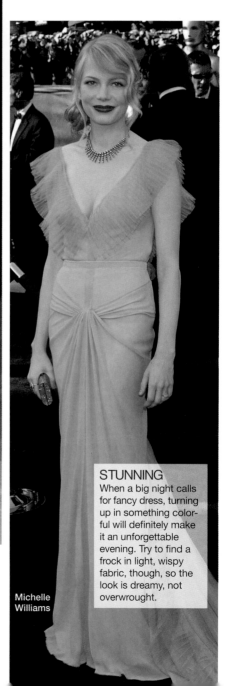

SIMPLE
If your desire is to go for peacock-worthy tints like neons, choose a lean, pared-down piece. You need to balance the bright with a more basic-shaped dress.

Reese Witherspoon

SEXY
If you want to be a traffic stopper, go full force in an eye-catching hue *and* eye-catching cut. But be prepared to get lots of attention.

Madonna

STUNNING
When a big night calls for fancy dress, turning up in something color-ful will definitely make it an unforgettable evening. Try to find a frock in light, wispy fabric, though, so the look is dreamy, not overwrought.

Michelle Williams

"If you like color, don't hold back. The bolder you go, the younger the attitude." —ISAAC MIZRAHI

GET THE LOOK

Night Brights

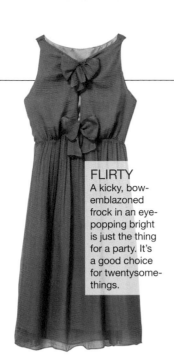

FLIRTY
A kicky, bow-emblazoned frock in an eye-popping bright is just the thing for a party. It's a good choice for twentysome-things.

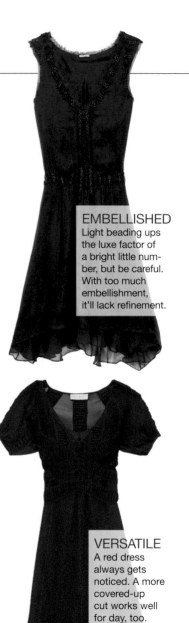

EMBELLISHED
Light beading ups the luxe factor of a bright little num-ber, but be careful. With too much embellishment, it'll lack refinement.

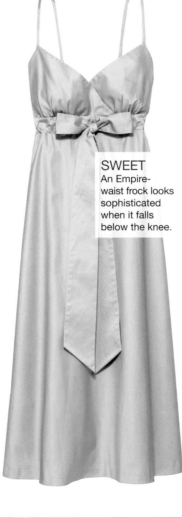

SWEET
An Empire-waist frock looks sophisticated when it falls below the knee.

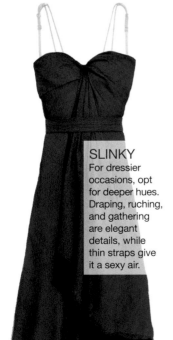

SLINKY
For dressier occasions, opt for deeper hues. Draping, ruching, and gathering are elegant details, while thin straps give it a sexy air.

VERSATILE
A red dress always gets noticed. A more covered-up cut works well for day, too.

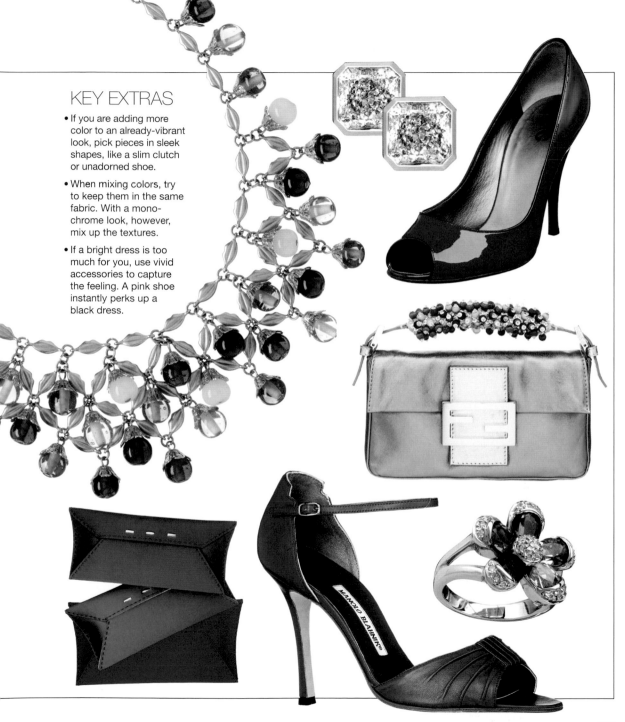

KEY EXTRAS

- If you are adding more color to an already-vibrant look, pick pieces in sleek shapes, like a slim clutch or unadorned shoe.

- When mixing colors, try to keep them in the same fabric. With a monochrome look, however, mix up the textures.

- If a bright dress is too much for you, use vivid accessories to capture the feeling. A pink shoe instantly perks up a black dress.

After-Sundown Sparkle

Metallics and sequins are all about glitz and glamour—perfect for spotlight-seeking style setters

Come nightfall, some of us just want to be the star of the show. And the best way to shine is to, well, shine. Slinky silver fabrics, glimmering gold, shimmering sequins, and razzle-dazzle rhinestones will turn any dress into something special. Be cautious, though; there is a fine line between tasteful and tacky when it comes to lamé fabrics and ornate embellishment. If there is so much beading on a frock that it's weighing you down, you've probably gone too far. Ditto if the look recalls the disco era. Keep it fresh and modern with slim silhouettes, lightweight fabrics, and solid or single-tone looks. And when your dress is bejeweled, go easy with your accessories. There's no need for a showy necklace or earrings when your outfit is already twinkling. Toned-down hair and makeup are also a good way to keep a sparkly look in check.

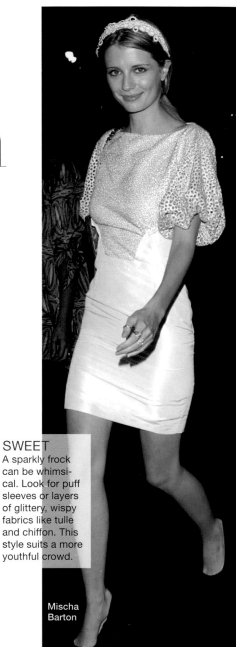

SWEET
A sparkly frock can be whimsical. Look for puff sleeves or layers of glittery, wispy fabrics like tulle and chiffon. This style suits a more youthful crowd.

Mischa Barton

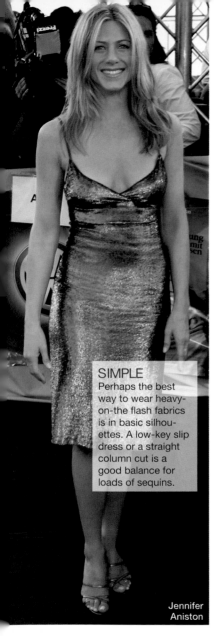

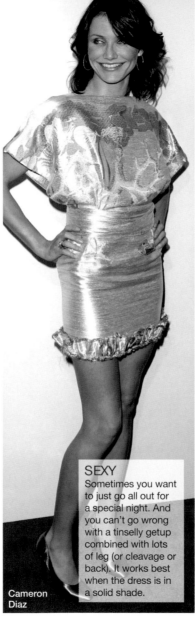

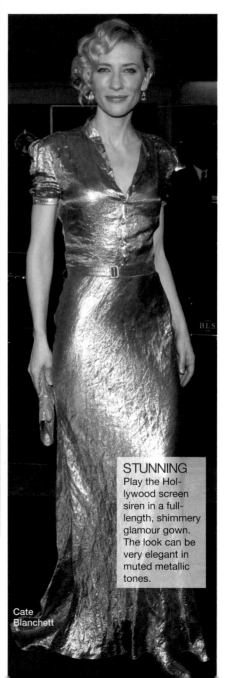

SIMPLE
Perhaps the best way to wear heavy-on-the flash fabrics is in basic silhouettes. A low-key slip dress or a straight column cut is a good balance for loads of sequins.

Jennifer Aniston

SEXY
Sometimes you want to just go all out for a special night. And you can't go wrong with a tinselly getup combined with lots of leg (or cleavage or back). It works best when the dress is in a solid shade.

Cameron Diaz

STUNNING
Play the Hollywood screen siren in a full-length, shimmery glamour gown. The look can be very elegant in muted metallic tones.

Cate Blanchett

"Sexy clothes are always relevant, because they are empowering."
—ZAC POSEN

GET THE LOOK

After-Sundown Sparkle

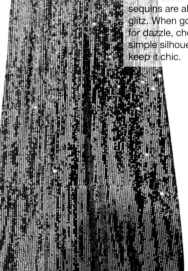

FLIRTY
A sequined mini will make a splash at any soiree. Too short for you? Try it with jeans or slim pants.

DANCEWORTHY
Gold lamé says dancing on the table. A frock with short sleeves and a covered-up neckline stops it from seeming crass.

ULTRAGLAM
Full-on silver or gold sequins are all about glitz. When going for dazzle, choose a simple silhouette to keep it chic.

FLASHY
A coatdress can be a flattering way to get in on the shiny, sparkly style without revealing too much. Pick a coat in a lighter fabric for the most becoming look.

SOPHISTICATED
Metallics and sequins can be toned down. Try them on separates for just a hint of shimmer.

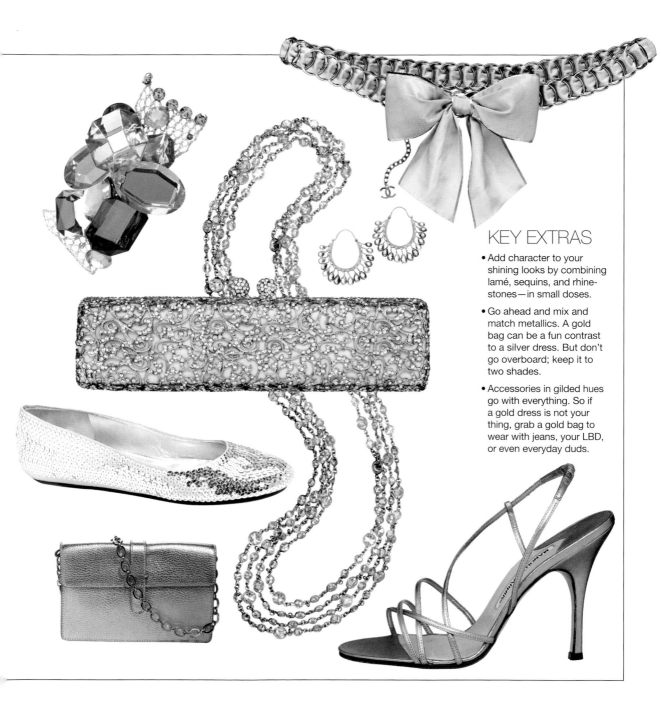

KEY EXTRAS

- Add character to your shining looks by combining lamé, sequins, and rhinestones—in small doses.

- Go ahead and mix and match metallics. A gold bag can be a fun contrast to a silver dress. But don't go overboard; keep it to two shades.

- Accessories in gilded hues go with everything. So if a gold dress is not your thing, grab a gold bag to wear with jeans, your LBD, or even everyday duds.

The Tuxedo

A man's black-tie standard gets a sexy, sophisticated spin as a woman's soiree-worthy evening ensemble

Dressing up is not necessarily all about the dress. The right two-piece ensemble can be just as sexy as any frock. Take the classic French evening suit *le smoking:* It oozes sex appeal, especially when worn with a slinky camisole (or nothing at all) underneath. A sleek men's-style tux is the ideal option if you're not willing to bare all in a wispy dress. The traditional black-and-white pairing is always dramatic, and the simplicity of the suit allows you to transform it at your whim. Wearing a lacy bra that peeks out from under the jacket is coy and sultry; a high-neck, ruffle-front blouse gives the look a retro spin; and swapping the conventional tuxedo pants for a superskinny leather or denim pair lends a fashion-forward flair. Plus, changing up your underpinnings and pairings can take the ensemble from dinner appropriate to cocktails to a formal affair. The very best part about wearing a tuxedo at night is it can hide everything, reveal a little, or show a lot—whichever look you choose!

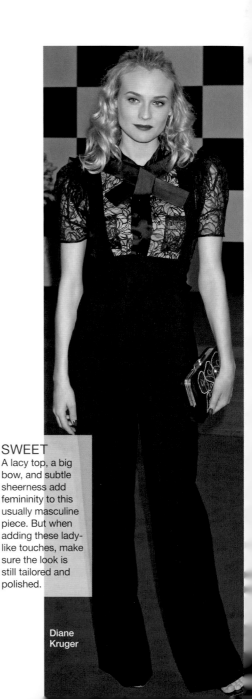

SWEET
A lacy top, a big bow, and subtle sheerness add femininity to this usually masculine piece. But when adding these lady-like touches, make sure the look is still tailored and polished.

Diane Kruger

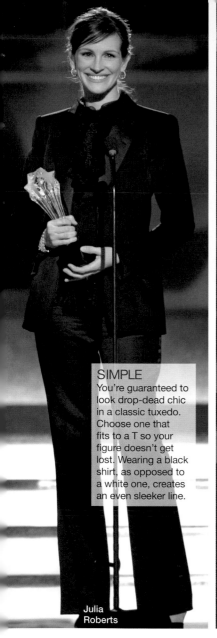

SIMPLE
You're guaranteed to look drop-dead chic in a classic tuxedo. Choose one that fits to a T so your figure doesn't get lost. Wearing a black shirt, as opposed to a white one, creates an even sleeker line.

Julia Roberts

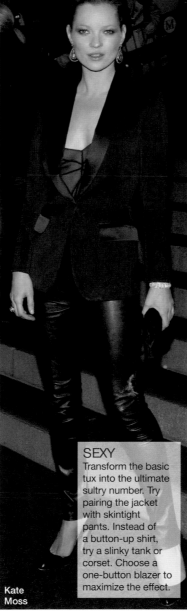

SEXY
Transform the basic tux into the ultimate sultry number. Try pairing the jacket with skintight pants. Instead of a button-up shirt, try a slinky tank or corset. Choose a one-button blazer to maximize the effect.

Kate Moss

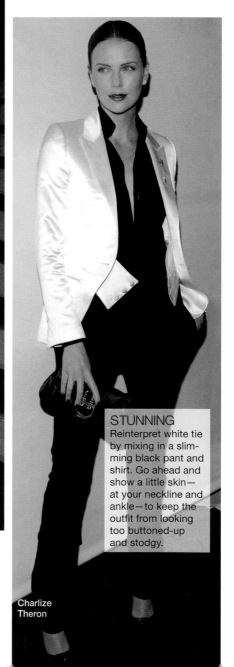

STUNNING
Reinterpret white tie by mixing in a slimming black pant and shirt. Go ahead and show a little skin—at your neckline and ankle—to keep the outfit from looking too buttoned-up and stodgy.

Charlize Theron

"A tux is perhaps the more sophisticated option." —GIORGIO ARMANI

GET THE LOOK

The Tuxedo

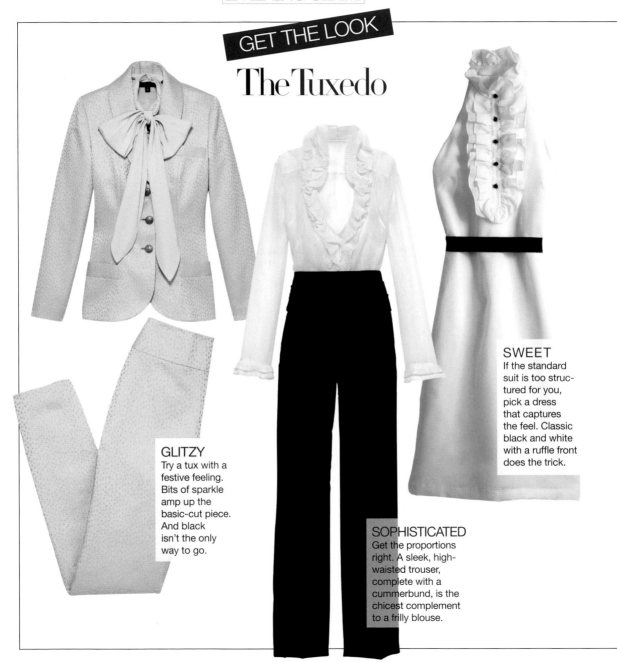

GLITZY
Try a tux with a
festive feeling.
Bits of sparkle
amp up the
basic-cut piece.
And black
isn't the only
way to go.

SOPHISTICATED
Get the proportions
right. A sleek, high-
waisted trouser,
complete with a
cummerbund, is the
chicest complement
to a frilly blouse.

SWEET
If the standard
suit is too struc-
tured for you,
pick a dress
that captures
the feel. Classic
black and white
with a ruffle front
does the trick.

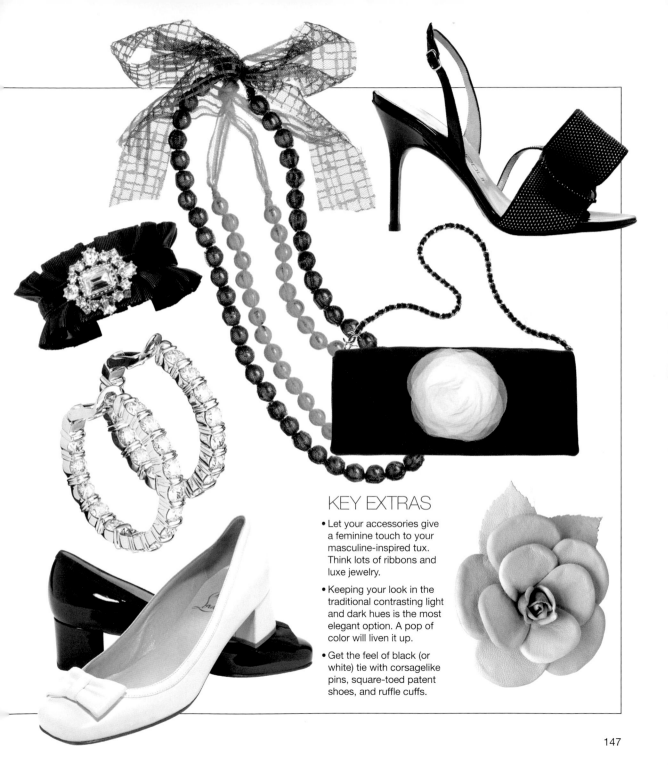

KEY EXTRAS

- Let your accessories give a feminine touch to your masculine-inspired tux. Think lots of ribbons and luxe jewelry.

- Keeping your look in the traditional contrasting light and dark hues is the most elegant option. A pop of color will liven it up.

- Get the feel of black (or white) tie with corsagelike pins, square-toed patent shoes, and ruffle cuffs.

The Perfect Dress for Your Shape

There is a dress out there to suit all body types. Find the cut that works best for you.

Everyone should have a go-to cocktail dress, whether it's the one you grab when you have an unexpected date, the piece you toss in your suitcase on every trip, or the sexy number you know your husband loves. The most important element in seeking out your ever-reliable frock is fit. Luckily, dresses today come in many cuts, so there is inevitably one that is most flattering for your figure. Once you discover the style that looks best on you, stick with it and you'll always feel confident.

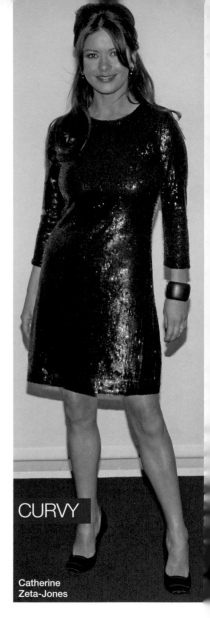

CURVY

Catherine Zeta-Jones

An A-line construction will give you a slender line.
Whether your frock has long or short sleeves or none at all, pick a trim, tailored, but not too tight cut. Stay away from anything baggy. It'll make your womanly figure look matronly.

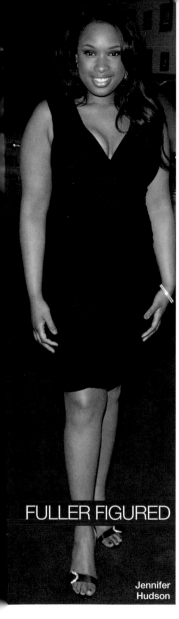

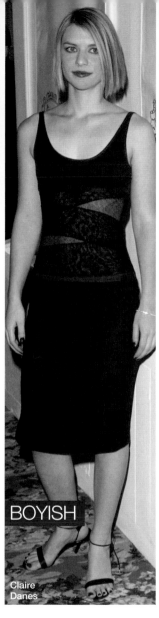

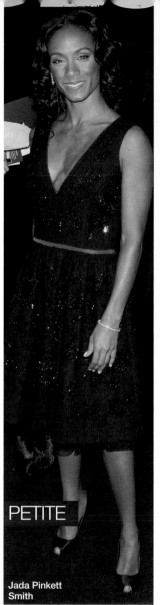

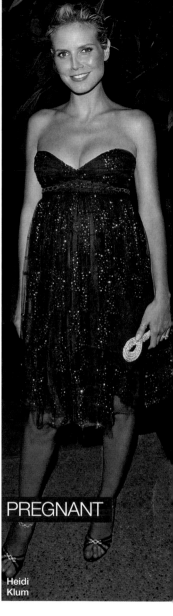

FULLER FIGURED

Jennifer Hudson

BOYISH

Claire Danes

PETITE

Jada Pinkett Smith

PREGNANT

Heidi Klum

You'd be surprised how well draping, pliable jersey, and other soft fabrics can work for you. Manipulate them around your figure—always tight around the waist. Remember, showing skin in strategic spots detracts from other places.

A formfitting frock is the way to go, especially if there is extra detailing around the waist—an important spot to emphasize. A simple tank reveals a decent amount of skin, giving your look a feminine air while still maintaining elegance.

Just because you are small framed doesn't mean you have to shun volume. While slip-of-a-thing frocks always work, a fuller silhouette with a well-defined waist can, too. The key is to balance, say, a swingy skirt with a fitted, more scantily cut top.

Work around your baby bump. That means focus on the waist, even if it is right under your bust. Empire lines can be your best friend during this time. Strapless styles look sweet if you can keep your bust safely in place.

Dressed-Down
Dress-Up

Sometimes your after-dark activities are low-key—but that doesn't mean you don't want to look gorgeous

Not every evening out is a big to-do requiring hours of primping. Most of the time, you're going to dinner with friends, out on dates, or entertaining at home. A full-on party look may not be necessary, but you still want to look special and different from your everyday style. So, how to look fancy but not formal? There are a handful of looks that best reveal the sexy-casual-cool combo. From a slinky top with basic pants to a touch of shine paired with something simple, casual evening looks can be easy to pull off.

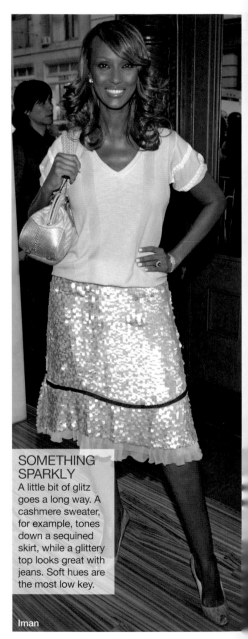

SOMETHING SPARKLY
A little bit of glitz goes a long way. A cashmere sweater, for example, tones down a sequined skirt, while a glittery top looks great with jeans. Soft hues are the most low key.

Iman

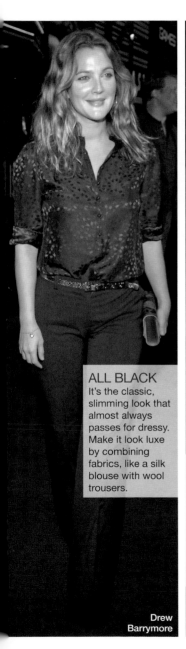

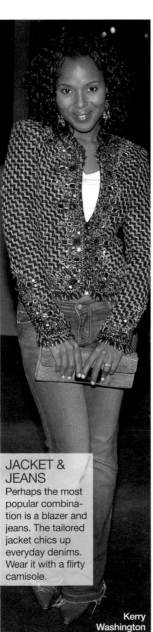

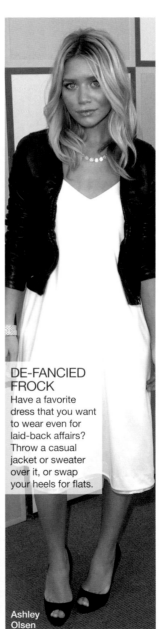

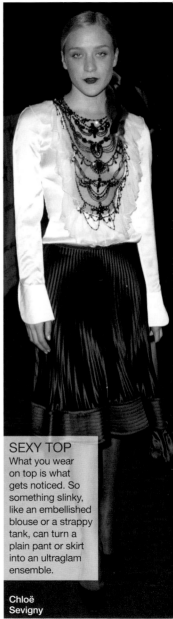

ALL BLACK

It's the classic, slimming look that almost always passes for dressy. Make it look luxe by combining fabrics, like a silk blouse with wool trousers.

JACKET & JEANS

Perhaps the most popular combination is a blazer and jeans. The tailored jacket chics up everyday denims. Wear it with a flirty camisole.

DE-FANCIED FROCK

Have a favorite dress that you want to wear even for laid-back affairs? Throw a casual jacket or sweater over it, or swap your heels for flats.

SEXY TOP

What you wear on top is what gets noticed. So something slinky, like an embellished blouse or a strappy tank, can turn a plain pant or skirt into an ultraglam ensemble.

Drew Barrymore

Kerry Washington

Ashley Olsen

Chloë Sevigny

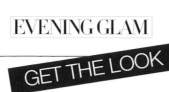

From Office...

Dashing from your desk to post-work drinks? Leave the serious look behind and switch it up for something sexy.

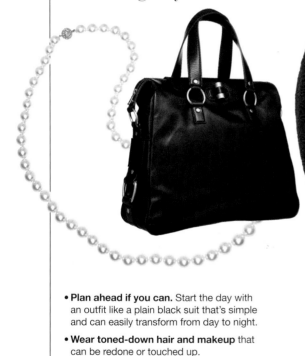

- **Plan ahead if you can.** Start the day with an outfit like a plain black suit that's simple and can easily transform from day to night.

- **Wear toned-down hair and makeup** that can be redone or touched up.

- **Wear a button-up**—or anything that slips off with ease and doesn't mess up your hair and makeup, as you'll no doubt have to make a quick switch.

- **Carry a tote** that morning that's big enough to hold the pieces you'll change into at the end of the day.

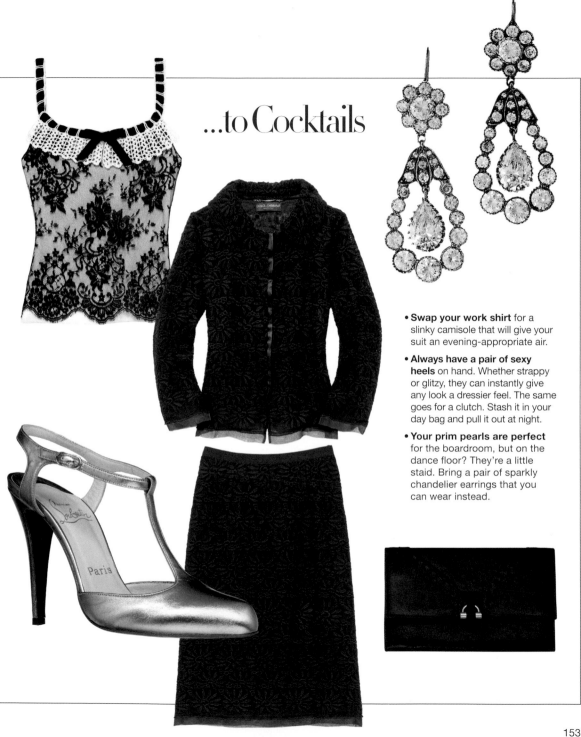

...to Cocktails

- **Swap your work shirt** for a slinky camisole that will give your suit an evening-appropriate air.

- **Always have a pair of sexy heels** on hand. Whether strappy or glitzy, they can instantly give any look a dressier feel. The same goes for a clutch. Stash it in your day bag and pull it out at night.

- **Your prim pearls are perfect** for the boardroom, but on the dance floor? They're a little staid. Bring a pair of sparkly chandelier earrings that you can wear instead.

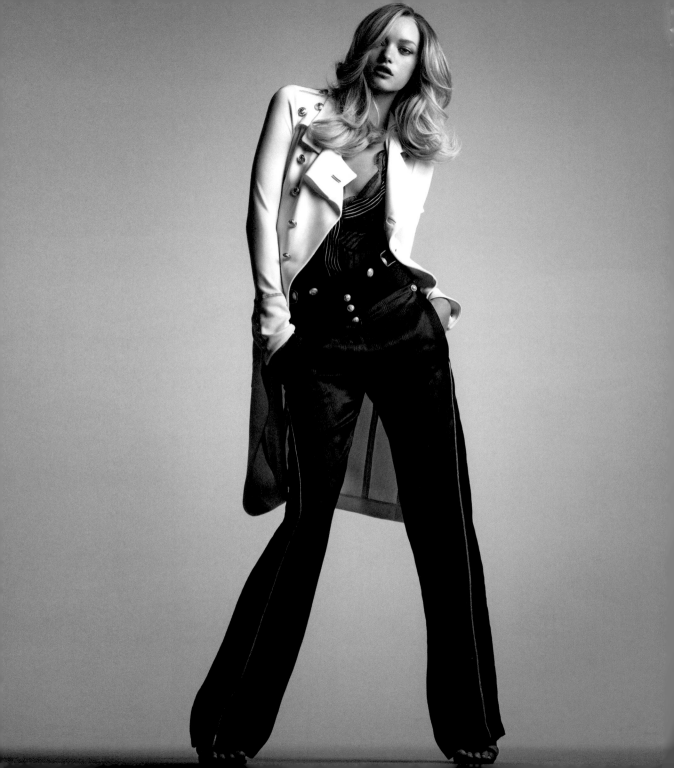

Casual Chic

7. Look polished and pulled together every day

"Style is primarily a matter of instinct."
—BILL BLASS

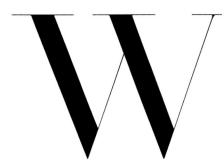

When we're not putting on a power look for the office or gussying up for a special affair, dressing is easy, right? Well, sometimes it's more difficult to pull yourself together when there *isn't* a dress code. Casual days are often the times when you have the most freedom and when fashion rules (dated or not) generally don't apply; there are no standards, no uniforms, and no obvious requirements. But that means you have lots of choices—and assembling a look is all in your hands. Not only do you get to wear exactly what you want and like, you also have a great opportunity to let your true personal style shine. Whether you are meeting your friends for lunch, out shopping, or spending the afternoon with your significant other, you want to look good, chic, and, most important, like yourself. And since getting dressed on your day off means you can mix and match to your heart's content, it's necessary to have a selection of the right pieces. They need to be versatile, have an air of refinement, and, above all, be comfortable.

Key Pieces

The essential elements to a great dressed-down wardrobe

1. Layering pieces are fundamental. Whether your low-key look of choice is a simple white tee, two tanks at a time, or a turtleneck tucked under your sweater, have stacks of them in different styles and fabric weights. They can be the basis for nearly any outfit.

2. Cozy up to knits. Sweaters, in all shapes and sizes, are comfy must-haves for weekends. Most of the time, they couldn't be easier to wear; pull one on atop pants—from jeans to trousers—and you're good to go.

3. Jackets bring everything together. And we're not talking about a stuffy suit blazer. There are plenty of casual styles that will add refinement to your dressed-down ensembles.

4. Jeans are everyone's favorite. No doubt the minute the weekend hits, you step into your beloved blues. Consider a variety of cuts, from wide leg and high waisted to skinny and cropped. You can create looks to suit every mood.

5. A casual coat should be adaptable and multipurpose. Unless you can afford to have a closetful, choose one for each season that can work with most of your clothes.

> "I tend to dress casually most of the time. I like to be comfortable, but I also like to have a bit of flair." —CAMERON DIAZ

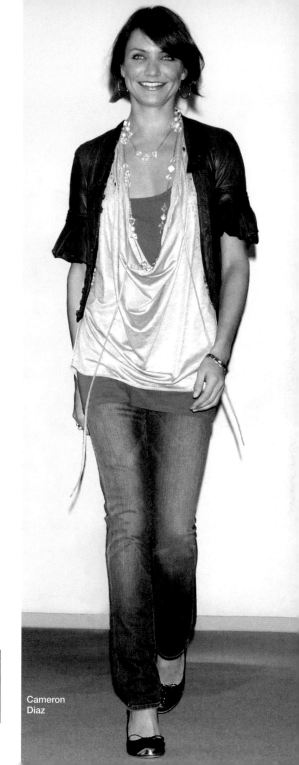

Cameron Diaz

Tees, Tanks & Turtlenecks

These basics are the ultimate in ease and versatility. No wonder we wear them so often.

We all live in tees. We wear them to the gym, to bed, and as undershirts; they are lifelong staples. But they don't have to be your brother's, husband's, or boyfriend's hand-me-downs. These soft cotton essentials are the building blocks of a casual wardrobe, not necessarily just around-the-house pieces. Today, T-shirts come in endless incarnations, and many of them are nice enough to wear on their own—out of the house. The best part is that they add such flexibility to your wardrobe. You can double up your tanks for an edgy and more substantial style or layer a turtleneck under your frock to give it a more covered-up (and warm) feel. Find a variety of cuts and colors and stock up!

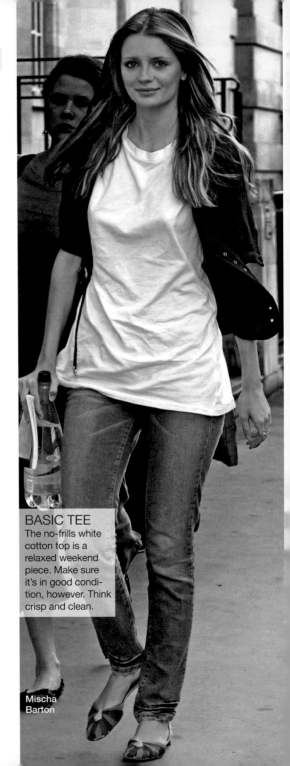

BASIC TEE
The no-frills white cotton top is a relaxed weekend piece. Make sure it's in good condition, however. Think crisp and clean.

Mischa Barton

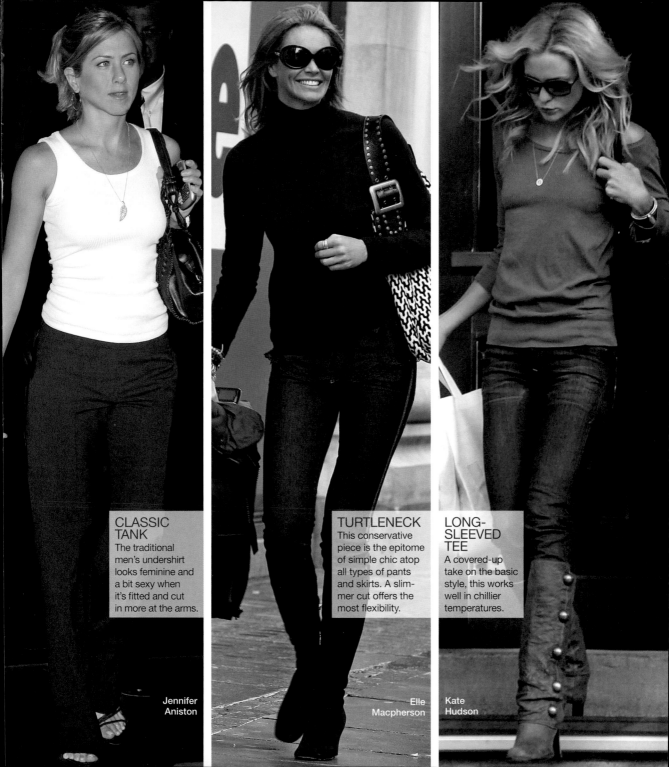

CLASSIC TANK

The traditional men's undershirt looks feminine and a bit sexy when it's fitted and cut in more at the arms.

Jennifer Aniston

TURTLENECK

This conservative piece is the epitome of simple chic atop all types of pants and skirts. A slimmer cut offers the most flexibility.

Elle Macpherson

LONG-SLEEVED TEE

A covered-up take on the basic style, this works well in chillier temperatures.

Kate Hudson

CASUAL CHIC

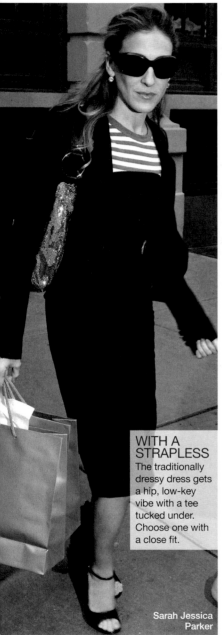

WITH A STRAPLESS
The traditionally dressy dress gets a hip, low-key vibe with a tee tucked under. Choose one with a close fit.

Sarah Jessica Parker

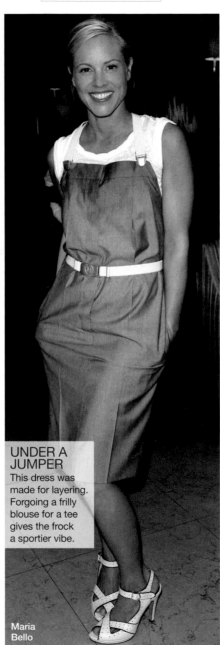

UNDER A JUMPER
This dress was made for layering. Forgoing a frilly blouse for a tee gives the frock a sportier vibe.

Maria Bello

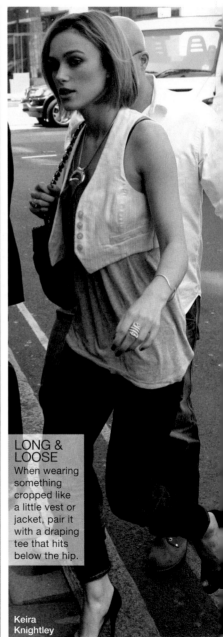

LONG & LOOSE
When wearing something cropped like a little vest or jacket, pair it with a draping tee that hits below the hip.

Keira Knightley

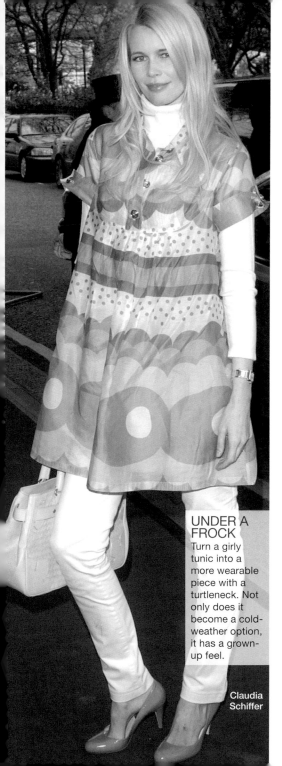

How to Wear It:
Tees, Tanks & Turtlenecks

- **Stick with longer styles.** Anything that hits at the hip or below has the most flexibility in what you can wear with it. Besides, a short tee that shows your midriff is a touch uncouth.

- **Pay attention to the weight of the fabric.** If it's thin and a little sheer, it's best worn under something or doubled up with another piece. Pick a slightly weightier style when wearing it alone so it's not indecent.

- **Layering gives new life to your dresses.** A springy frock can be worn well into fall when paired with a tee, tank, or turtleneck. Try it with your sundresses, shirtdresses, jumpers, and the like. Don't be afraid of the unconventional. For example, a T-shirt can take a strapless dress from slinky to sporty.

- **Putting jersey tops under your dresses** tones down the sexiness, making revealing numbers more appropriate for conservative environments like the office.

- **Don't go too loose when layering with dresses.** If your top is baggy, it won't lie properly and will look sloppy. Thin and fitted tees are best as underpinnings.

- **Slouchy cuts look great** under jackets and vests. Look for pieces that have a little movement and don't hug your hips in an unflattering way.

- **The key to looking smart in a tee** is to wear a clean and fresh one. Have one stack for working out and one for wearing out, and don't mix them. And know when to let go. If it's yellowed and holey, trash it. You may think no one will notice the difference ... but they will!

Knits

Cozy and comfortable sweaters of all styles are wardrobe mainstays

Are you the type of person who dreams of snuggling up in a soft sweater in front of a fire once the leaves start to change? Do you put on your favorite chunky cashmere turtleneck at the first sign of snow? Do you always have a cardie on hand, even in the dead of summer? Most of us rely on knits—thick or thin, embellished or classic, playful or refined—for practical purposes. But woollies should not be reserved for weekends in. They can pull together your look. Plus, they make for great cover-ups and transition pieces. A warm-weather frock, for example, instantly gets a fall feel when topped with a weighty wrap sweater, a soft alternative to a jacket or coat. Even on warm days, you'll benefit from having a little knit on hand to throw over your shoulders when going into overly air-conditioned environments. The best part about knits is how easy they can be. Throw on a V-neck with your favorite jeans and boots and, voilà, you've got an outfit.

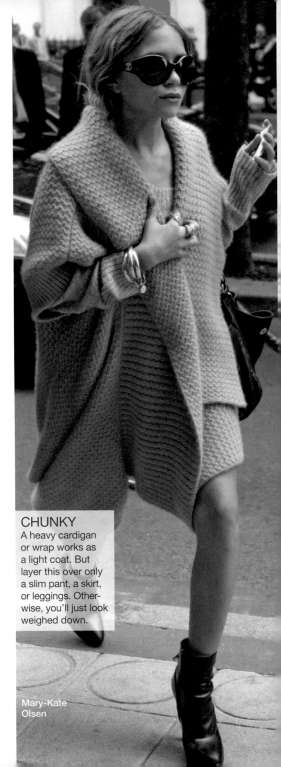

CHUNKY
A heavy cardigan or wrap works as a light coat. But layer this over only a slim pant, a skirt, or leggings. Otherwise, you'll just look weighed down.

Mary-Kate Olsen

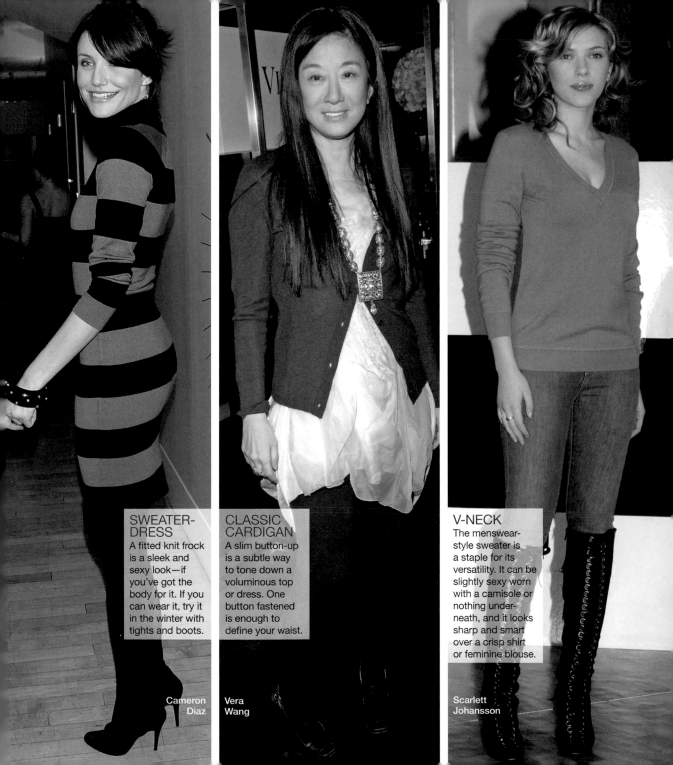

SWEATER-DRESS
A fitted knit frock is a sleek and sexy look—if you've got the body for it. If you can wear it, try it in the winter with tights and boots.

Cameron Diaz

CLASSIC CARDIGAN
A slim button-up is a subtle way to tone down a voluminous top or dress. One button fastened is enough to define your waist.

Vera Wang

V-NECK
The menswear-style sweater is a staple for its versatility. It can be slightly sexy worn with a camisole or nothing underneath, and it looks sharp and smart over a crisp shirt or feminine blouse.

Scarlett Johansson

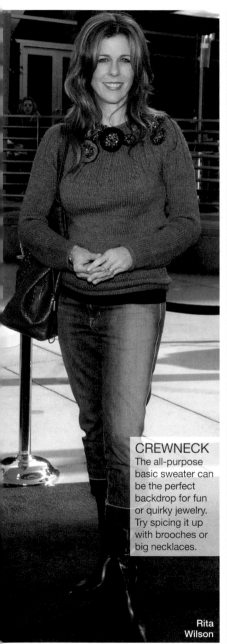

CREWNECK
The all-purpose basic sweater can be the perfect backdrop for fun or quirky jewelry. Try spicing it up with brooches or big necklaces.

Rita Wilson

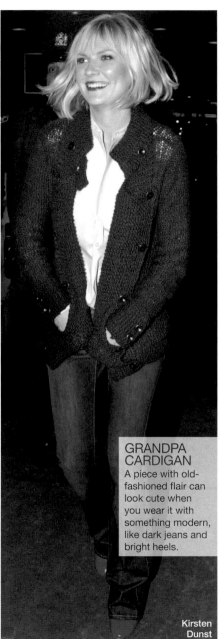

GRANDPA CARDIGAN
A piece with old-fashioned flair can look cute when you wear it with something modern, like dark jeans and bright heels.

Kirsten Dunst

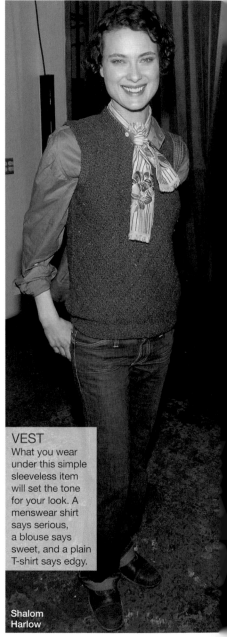

VEST
What you wear under this simple sleeveless item will set the tone for your look. A menswear shirt says serious, a blouse says sweet, and a plain T-shirt says edgy.

Shalom Harlow

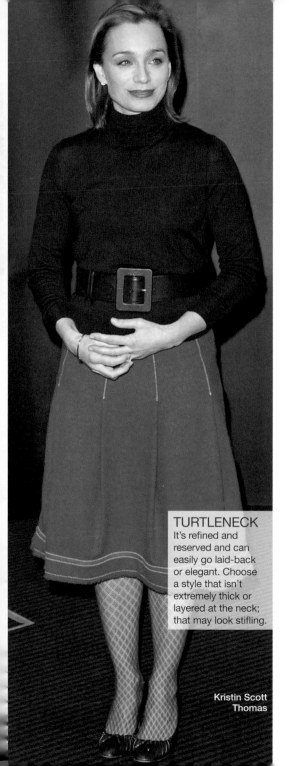

Kristin Scott
Thomas

How to Wear It:
Knits

- **Be open to new ways of styling sweaters.** They have become superchic wardrobe essentials. Pair turtlenecks with a full or pencil skirt (consider this for the office or evenings out), put a slightly loose-fitting boyfriend V-neck over a crisp white shirt worn with trousers, or pick a nearly sheer cashmere cardigan to go with a camisole and ball skirt.

- **The biggest risk you run** with these woolly tops is adding pounds. Battle the bulkiness with a belt—over thick and thin knits. Also, when wearing a cardigan, try leaving it open and belting your top underneath. That way your waist is defined, and your sweater is relaxed and easy.

- **Pay attention to where your sweater hits.** A piece that ends right above your hips can add thickness. Try slightly longer cuts that fall at midhip. In addition, think about clinginess. If your stomach is not so slim, a draped cut will lie nicely.

- **Consider what you wear underneath.** Stick with thin or light layers under your knits or just a smooth bra. Don't stuff a puff sleeve into the slim arm of a cardigan.

- **Let a chunky knit double as a jacket or coat.** Perfect for fall days or chilly summer nights, a sweater is a more laid-back and unstructured alternative.

- **Fabric counts.** Supersoft cashmere is always the most luxurious option. The more plies the better. It's a worthwhile investment, and if you take care of your cashmere knits, they'll last for years. Fine cottons are also great options for summer sweaters.

Jackets

Think beyond your basic blazer and there's a world of cover-up options out there

Whether cropped, long, fitted, or swingy, jackets are the ultimate finish to every outfit. Even if it's a casual weekend look, throwing a jacket on over your dress, atop your jeans, or with a skirt is an easy way to get just the right amount of polish. Forget notions of a stuffy formal jacket. (Save that for work if you must.) This piece comes in numerous styles, and there is certainly one out there to go with every look. Think about a cool leather cut, something edgy and fitted, a flared boho option, or a prim, ladylike piece. Remember, your jacket doesn't *have* to be a perfect match with your bottoms. In fact, a more casual piece offers greater flexibility. You should be able to wear it with denim, and even over a cocktail frock. The right jacket can be a complement to the rest of your ensemble, or it can be the centerpiece.

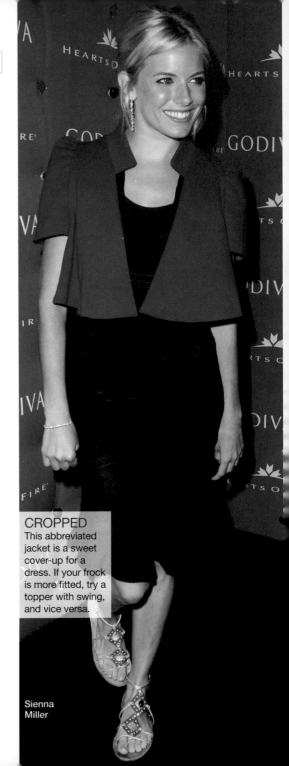

CROPPED
This abbreviated jacket is a sweet cover-up for a dress. If your frock is more fitted, try a topper with swing, and vice versa.

Sienna Miller

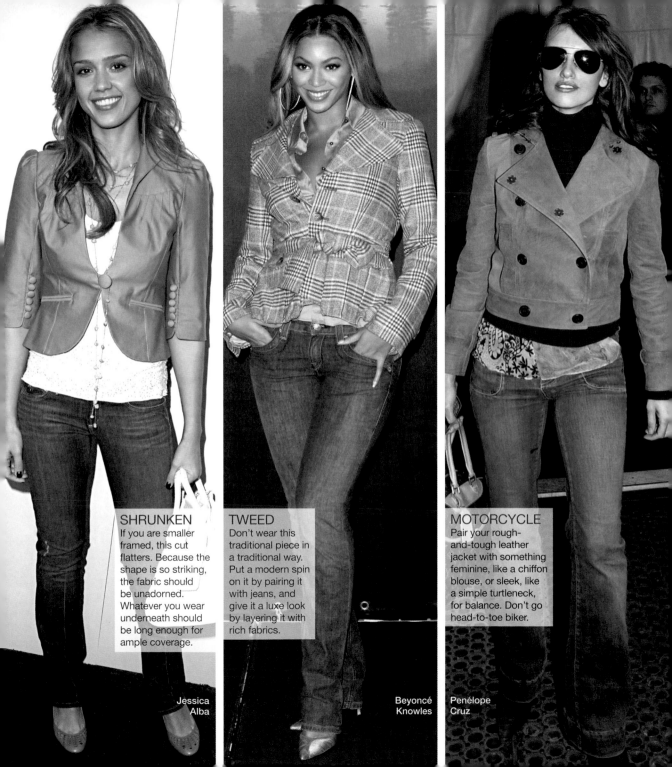

SHRUNKEN

If you are smaller framed, this cut flatters. Because the shape is so striking, the fabric should be unadorned. Whatever you wear underneath should be long enough for ample coverage.

TWEED

Don't wear this traditional piece in a traditional way. Put a modern spin on it by pairing it with jeans, and give it a luxe look by layering it with rich fabrics.

MOTORCYCLE

Pair your rough-and-tough leather jacket with something feminine, like a chiffon blouse, or sleek, like a simple turtleneck, for balance. Don't go head-to-toe biker.

Jessica Alba

Beyoncé Knowles

Penélope Cruz

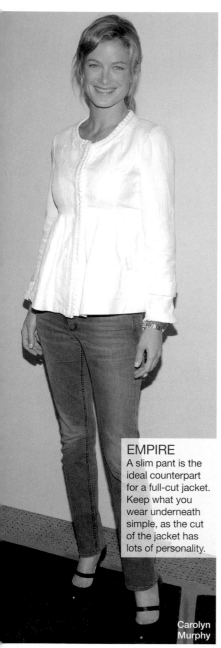

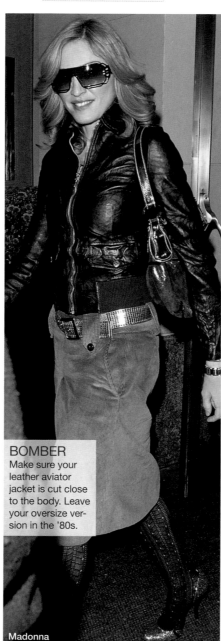

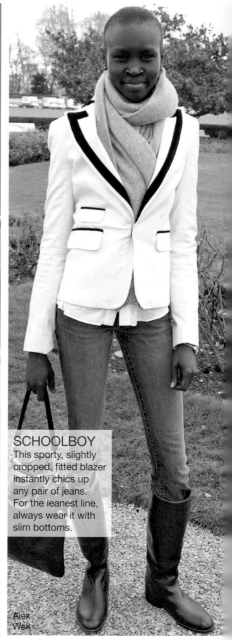

EMPIRE
A slim pant is the ideal counterpart for a full-cut jacket. Keep what you wear underneath simple, as the cut of the jacket has lots of personality.

Carolyn Murphy

BOMBER
Make sure your leather aviator jacket is cut close to the body. Leave your oversize version in the '80s.

Madonna

SCHOOLBOY
This sporty, slightly cropped, fitted blazer instantly chics up any pair of jeans. For the leanest line, always wear it with slim bottoms.

Alek Wek

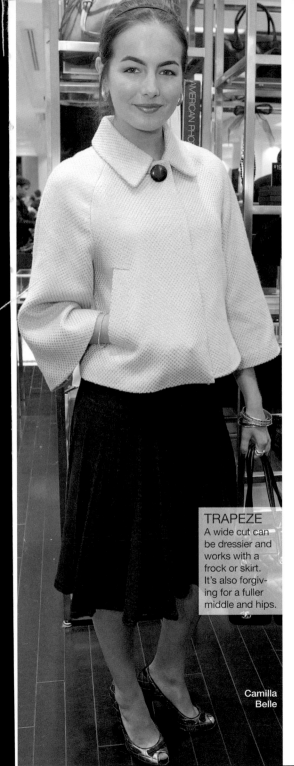

Camilla Belle

How to Wear It:
Jackets

- **Dress around your jacket.** Swapping one piece, such as a button-up shirt for a camisole, can change the ensemble's vibe.

- **Pay attention to proportion.** With a cropped jacket, for example, wear a longer shirt underneath or a high-waisted skirt or pant. It's okay if your top is longer than your jacket. In fact, it adds dimension to your look. The fuller your pant or skirt, the shorter or more fitted your jacket should be. A long, loose topper with, say, pleated trousers or a dirndl will just add pounds, and who wants that?

- **Mix it up.** Pair your jacket with an outfit of a contrasting style. An Empire-waist jacket gives a girly feel to skinny jeans, a tweedy style looks sweet with satin or velvet, and a leather piece can add a tough edge to a flirty frock.

- **Maintain a feminine silhouette.** Choose a piece that comes in at the waist, belt it, or pick a cropped cut that ends above your hips.

- **If you prefer a boxier cut,** try one that's shorter in length. And wear a fitted top underneath. Your jacket should add shape, not conceal it.

- **Don't overstuff.** Layering can look great, but too many tops, sweaters, and scarves underneath that jacket isn't flattering. If the buttons are pulling, shed a few layers or try a roomier cut.

Day Dresses

Flirty, boho, sexy, or demure—frocks should top your shopping list

If for any reason you hesitate when it comes to dresses for everyday wear—they're too girly, they show too much, or they're too fussy—it's time to think again. Yes, dresses can be overly feminine, reveal some leg, and sometimes seem tricky to wear, but they can also be sophisticated, refined, and beyond easy. In fact, they're a one-step wonder, and once you find a few cuts you like, you may not want to wear anything else. And you might be surprised to learn how flexible dresses can be. It's easier than you might expect to take an evening piece and make it appropriate for day (layering a tee underneath and swapping your heels for flats, for starters) or turn something slinky into something you can wear at work. (Try putting it over a tank top and wearing a structured jacket on top.) While dresses might be a tad pricier than separates, they are worth spending on. Wouldn't you pay a little extra on something that requires so little effort yet can look so chic?

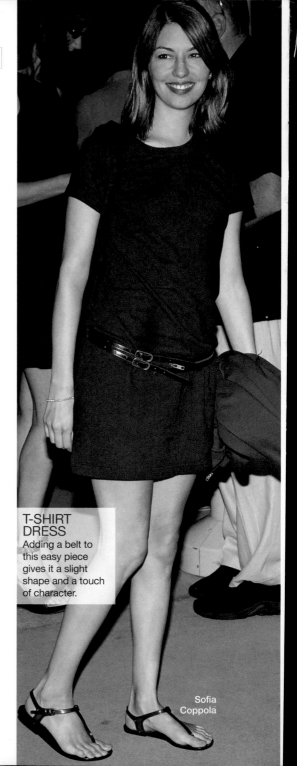

T-SHIRT DRESS
Adding a belt to this easy piece gives it a slight shape and a touch of character.

Sofia Coppola

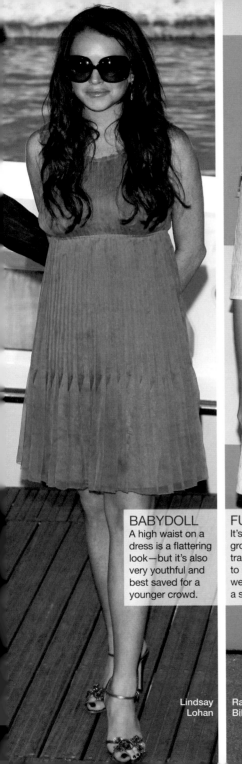

BABYDOLL
A high waist on a dress is a flattering look—but it's also very youthful and best saved for a younger crowd.

Lindsay Lohan

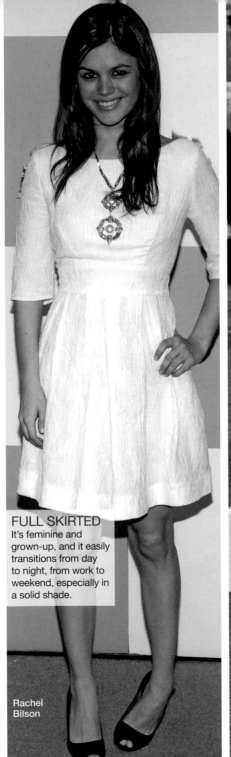

FULL SKIRTED
It's feminine and grown-up, and it easily transitions from day to night, from work to weekend, especially in a solid shade.

Rachel Bilson

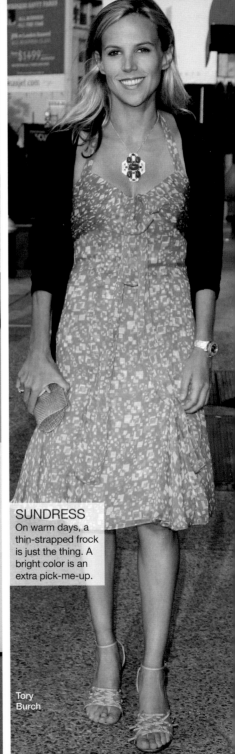

SUNDRESS
On warm days, a thin-strapped frock is just the thing. A bright color is an extra pick-me-up.

Tory Burch

CASUAL CHIC

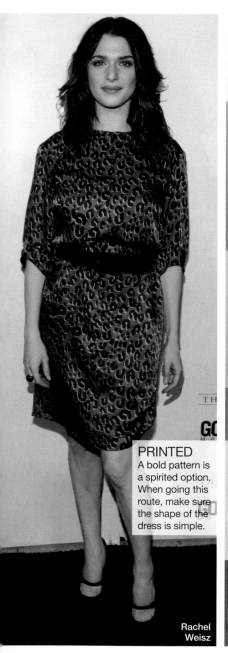

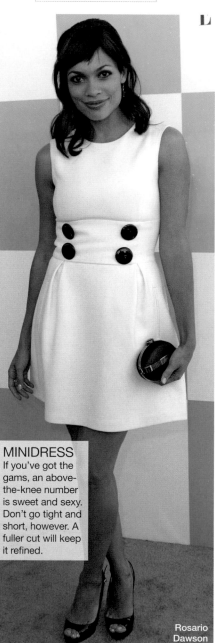

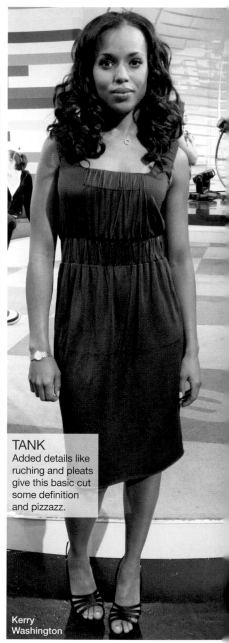

PRINTED
A bold pattern is a spirited option. When going this route, make sure the shape of the dress is simple.

MINIDRESS
If you've got the gams, an above-the-knee number is sweet and sexy. Don't go tight and short, however. A fuller cut will keep it refined.

TANK
Added details like ruching and pleats give this basic cut some definition and pizzazz.

Rachel Weisz

Rosario Dawson

Kerry Washington

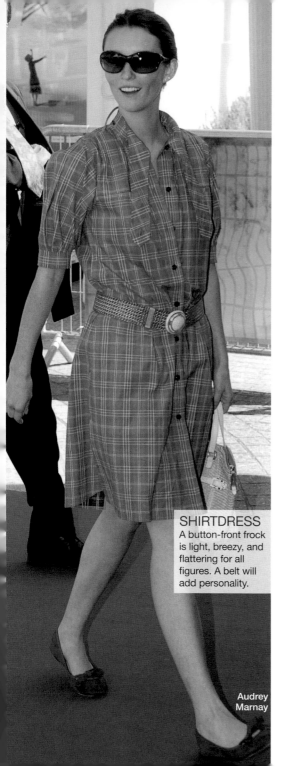

SHIRTDRESS
A button-front frock is light, breezy, and flattering for all figures. A belt will add personality.

Audrey Marnay

How to Wear It:
Day Dresses

- **While sundresses are a no-brainer** in the summer, you might hesitate before throwing on a frock on chillier days. But don't. A turtleneck or tee is the ideal underpinning, keeping you warm and letting your dress grab the attention it deserves. If you want more coverage, throw on a cardigan. Opaque tights, boots, or a chunky pump add to the transformative effect.

- **Most dresses can be very forgiving.** A full-skirted style can mask wide hips. But beware: Gypsy tiers often add unwanted volume. For the optimum flattering silhouette, select a piece that highlights your figure.

- **If choosing a piece with volume,** make sure it's balanced. A bubble-skirted frock, for example, should have a slim top, while a pouf-sleeved piece should be narrower on the bottom.

- **Don't get lost in the drape of a dress.** A cinched waist, a belt, a sash, or a nipped-in cut will keep your body looking its best.

- **Consider lengths, too.** A just-above-the-knee hem works well with most body types.

- **Ultrafeminine Empire-waist** and babydoll dresses can be a fun alternative to more conservative cuts but are not appropriate for more mature age groups.

- **Keep in mind that the higher your hemline,** the lower your heel. Wear minidresses with flats when going for a more casual look.

Jeans

We can't get enough of this all-American staple that goes with just about everything

On casual days, our good old blues are most likely the first piece we turn to. They are comfortable and easy, and there isn't much you *can't* wear them with. As your base, jeans allow you to get glammed up or go laid-back, edgy, rugged, or grungy—you name it. And it's not just about basic indigo hues. Jeans look great in shades of black, white, and gray, among others. That's the best part about denim: its transformative quality. And jeans have come a long way from just being weekend wear. They are acceptable nearly everywhere.

Many people wear them to work, and they're often okay in restaurants and even at cocktail parties. The only challenge lies in finding the perfect cut. Many of us have stacks of jeans but end up favoring one pair, because once we find the denim that looks best, that's all we want to wear.

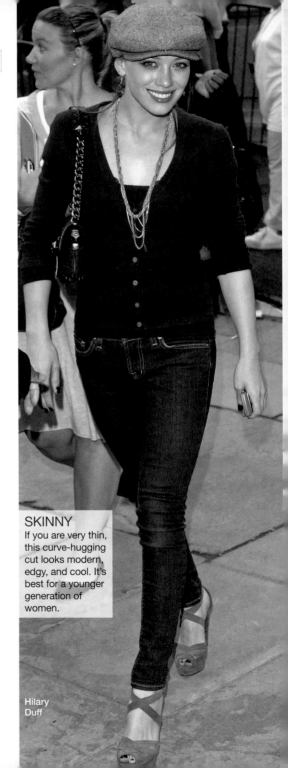

SKINNY
If you are very thin, this curve-hugging cut looks modern, edgy, and cool. It's best for a younger generation of women.

Hilary Duff

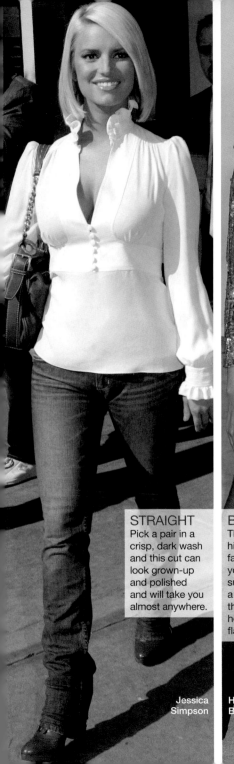

STRAIGHT
Pick a pair in a crisp, dark wash and this cut can look grown-up and polished and will take you almost anywhere.

Jessica Simpson

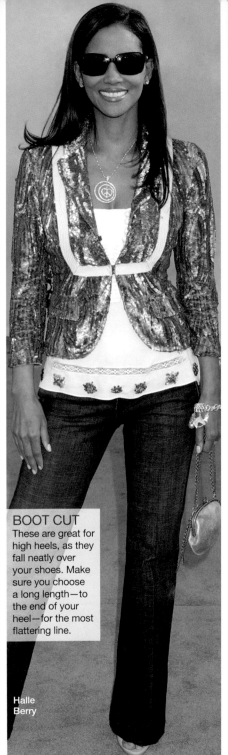

BOOT CUT
These are great for high heels, as they fall neatly over your shoes. Make sure you choose a long length—to the end of your heel—for the most flattering line.

Halle Berry

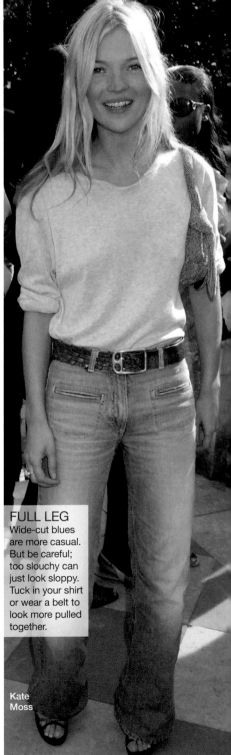

FULL LEG
Wide-cut blues are more casual. But be careful; too slouchy can just look sloppy. Tuck in your shirt or wear a belt to look more pulled together.

Kate Moss

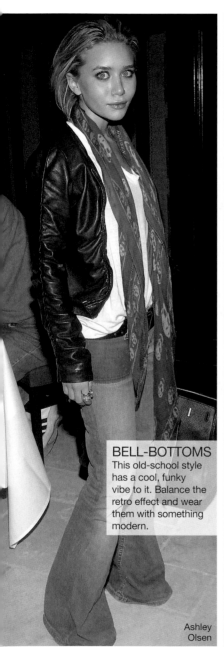

BELL-BOTTOMS
This old-school style has a cool, funky vibe to it. Balance the retro effect and wear them with something modern.

Ashley Olsen

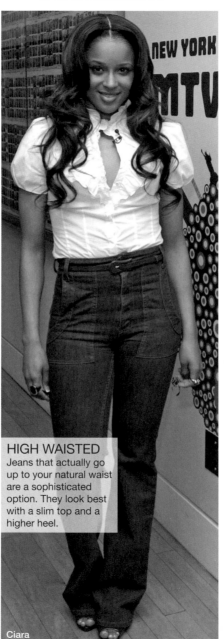

HIGH WAISTED
Jeans that actually go up to your natural waist are a sophisticated option. They look best with a slim top and a higher heel.

Ciara

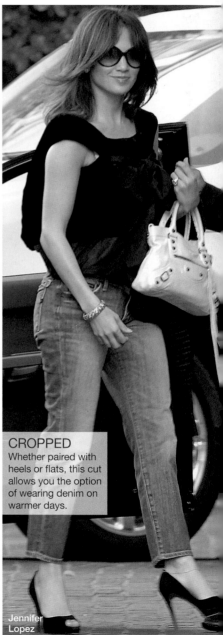

CROPPED
Whether paired with heels or flats, this cut allows you the option of wearing denim on warmer days.

Jennifer Lopez

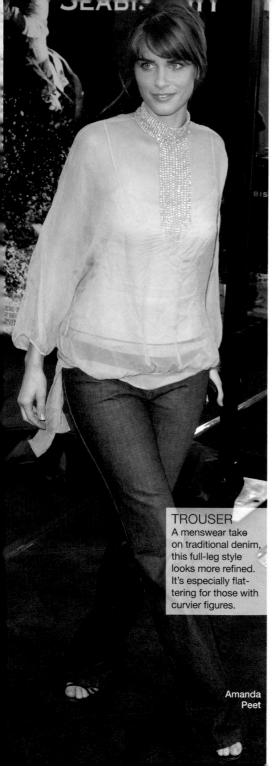

TROUSER
A menswear take on traditional denim, this full-leg style looks more refined. It's especially flattering for those with curvier figures.

Amanda Peet

How to Wear It:
Jeans

- **When shopping for jeans,** assess your lifestyle needs and buy accordingly. Do you wear them to the office? Saturdays only? Dressed up for evenings? Dark, clean washes look neat and more appropriate for evening. Worn-in, frayed jeans are best kept to casual days.

- **Heels? Flats? Both?** Consider what shoes you wear with your jeans. Buy cuts in different lengths. Have at least one pair of blues to wear with your ballet flats and one to wear with your stilettos.

- **Experiment with different styles.** There are countless styles of jeans out there, and you may feel overwhelmed to think of trying them all on. Don't be afraid to ask a salesperson for help. It's a good idea to put the time in initially. Then, once you find the perfect pair, buy in multiples if you can.

- **Tighter jeans often look sleeker.** Baggier, slouchier styles look more casual and aren't always as flattering. Plus, denim usually stretches as you wear it. So don't be afraid for go for a smaller size than you normally wear.

- **To tuck or not to tuck?** When it comes to boots and jeans, many of us can't figure out how to put the two together. Tucking your denim into your knee-highs can look very jet-set, and skinny jeans fit smoothly. Don't stuff a baggy cut in there.

- **To wear your jeans over your boots,** a boot-cut or fuller leg works best. It doesn't look good if your boots show noticeably through your jeans.

Coats

You can't go out without one, so choose a major statement maker

It's the piece you don't often buy on a whim. You carefully analyze the options, contemplate, and ask your friends and family (and everyone else in the store) before you put down the credit card. There is no getting around it: A coat is a serious investment, so you must choose wisely. You want your coat to be special—it is the first and last thing other people see—but also high quality and classic, as it needs to be a workhorse. Aside from being durable, it needs to go with the multiple functions of your wardrobe—all your casual, work, and evening looks. This holds true even with the most casual pieces. But forget the notion that a coat should be basic because you wear it every day. For just that reason, it should be anything but. Purchase something you love, that will make you giddy with excitement each time you put it on.

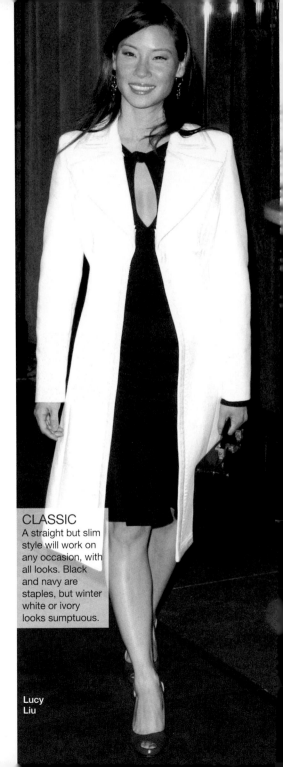

CLASSIC
A straight but slim style will work on any occasion, with all looks. Black and navy are staples, but winter white or ivory looks sumptuous.

Lucy
Liu

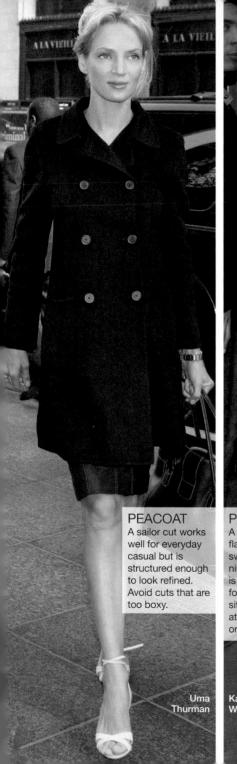

PEACOAT
A sailor cut works well for everyday casual but is structured enough to look refined. Avoid cuts that are too boxy.

Uma Thurman

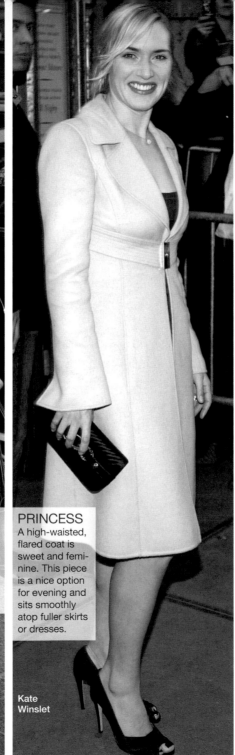

PRINCESS
A high-waisted, flared coat is sweet and feminine. This piece is a nice option for evening and sits smoothly atop fuller skirts or dresses.

Kate Winslet

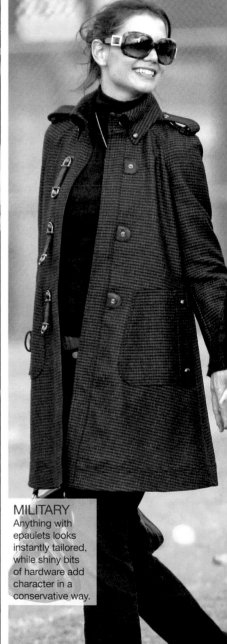

MILITARY
Anything with epaulets looks instantly tailored, while shiny bits of hardware add character in a conservative way.

Katie Holmes

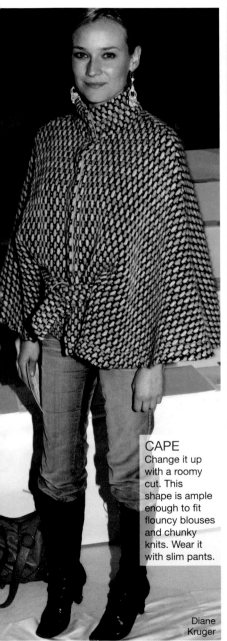

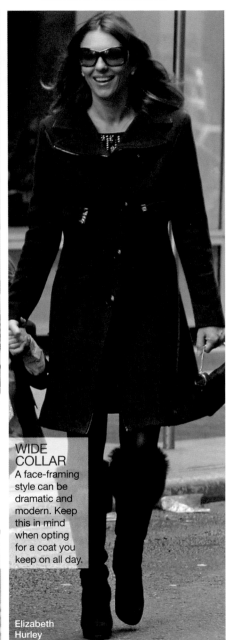

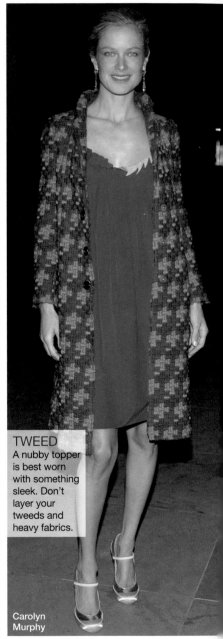

CAPE
Change it up with a roomy cut. This shape is ample enough to fit flouncy blouses and chunky knits. Wear it with slim pants.

WIDE COLLAR
A face-framing style can be dramatic and modern. Keep this in mind when opting for a coat you keep on all day.

TWEED
A nubby topper is best worn with something sleek. Don't layer your tweeds and heavy fabrics.

Diane Kruger

Elizabeth Hurley

Carolyn Murphy

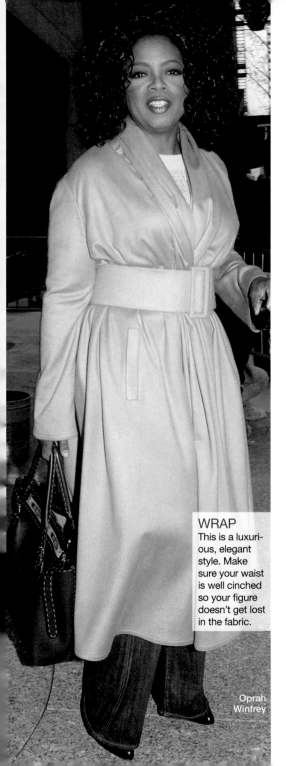

Oprah Winfrey

How to Wear It:
Coats

- **Because a coat is your outer layer,** the shape can make or break your look. A slim cut is, well, slimming. A style that's flared from the waist down works with full skirts but can often have too much volume for curvier figures.

- **For the most universally flattering look,** choose a piece that highlights the waist and is about knee length. Something nipped in at the waist is your best choice. If your coat is straight, cinch it with a regular wide belt.

- **If you can splurge on a second or third option,** consider a luxe coat, which can double as a dress. Pair it with pumps and opaque hose and you're cocktail ready.

- **In warmer months,** a lightweight coat looks refined and elegant over a dress. Pick one that matches for the most uptown air.

- **Soft-shoulder wrap styles** look luxurious and are cozy. Try them over tailored silhouettes.

- **Capes are a fun way to mix it up.** They're voluminous enough to handle lots of layering underneath.

- **For a more structured style,** a shiny-buttoned, belted military coat is a key piece, and it works well for the office.

- **The longer you go,** the more formal. Shorter styles are great for every day, while floor-sweeping cuts look elegant in the evening. A three-quarter length generally goes anywhere.

What's Your Weekend Style?

When the strict suit or fancy frock comes off, your low-key, laid-back style can flourish

Maybe every day at work you confidently strut in a skinny pencil skirt and a crisp button-up shirt. Perhaps your office uniform is jeans, a blouse, and a blazer. But on Saturday, you don't want to wear the structured looks you've been wearing all week. Most likely, you are putting on something much more comfortable. While your weekend look should be relaxed, it shouldn't be sloppy. If you're out shopping, running errands, or even at the movies, there is always the chance you'll bump into someone you know. We've all been there; suddenly we're embarrassed about our not-so-pulled-together look and scolding ourselves for not dressing just a little better. So now's the time to let yourself shine, even on the most casual of days. Weekend dressing is fun! Plus it's another chance to unleash your personal style.

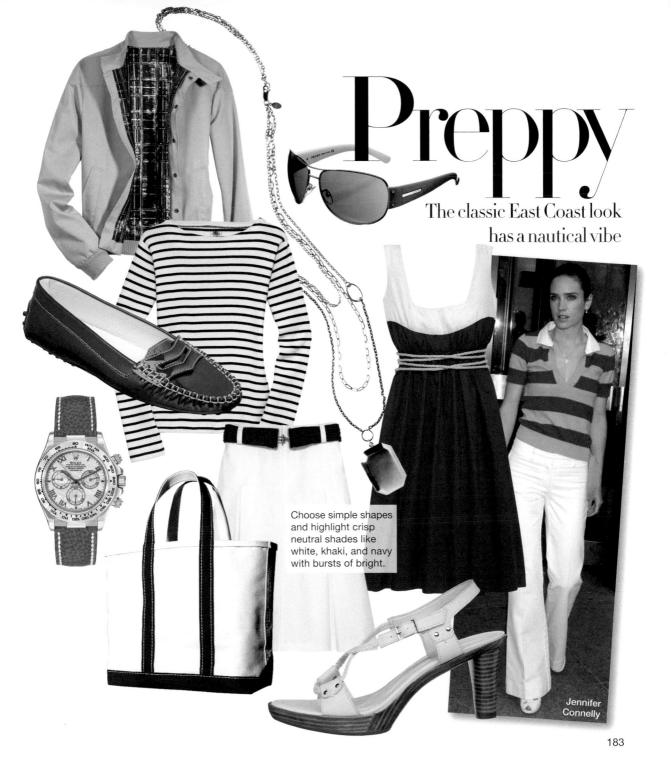

Preppy

The classic East Coast look has a nautical vibe

Choose simple shapes and highlight crisp neutral shades like white, khaki, and navy with bursts of bright.

Jennifer Connelly

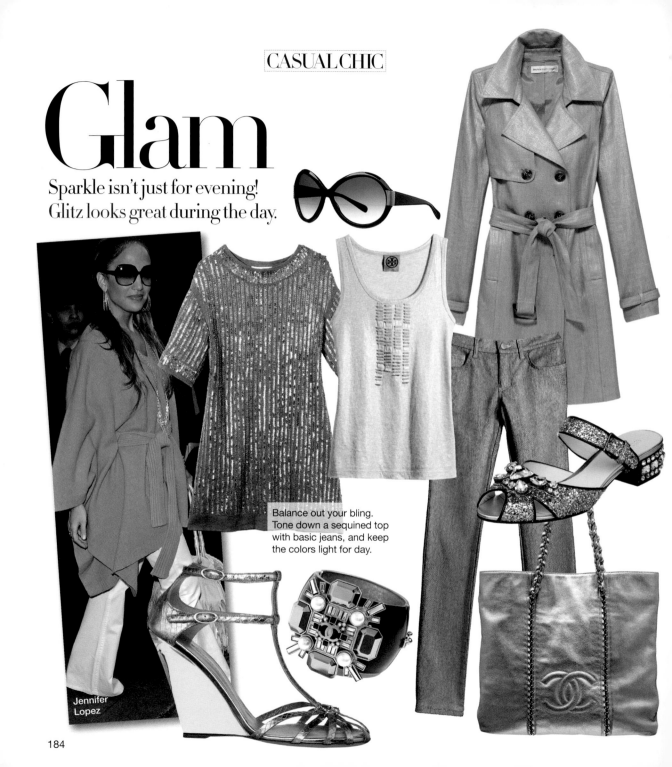

Glam

Sparkle isn't just for evening!
Glitz looks great during the day.

Balance out your bling. Tone down a sequined top with basic jeans, and keep the colors light for day.

Jennifer Lopez

184

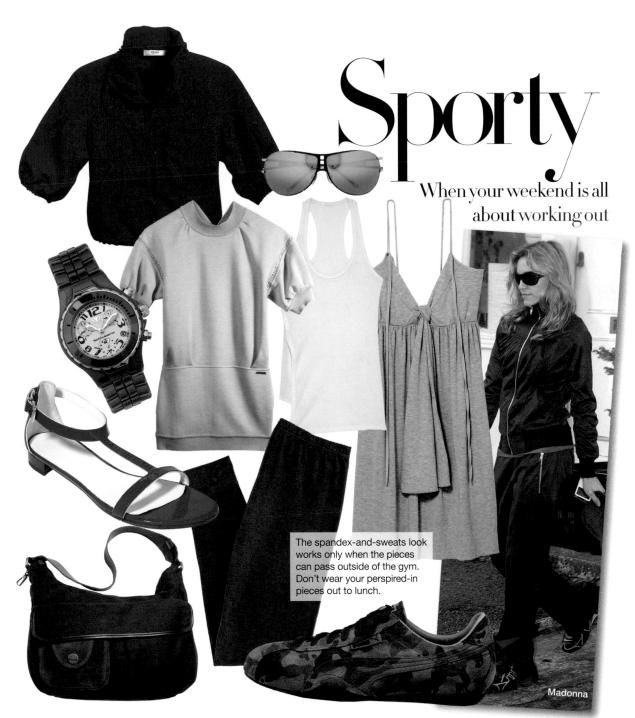

Sporty

When your weekend is all about working out

The spandex-and-sweats look works only when the pieces can pass outside of the gym. Don't wear your perspired-in pieces out to lunch.

Madonna

Urban

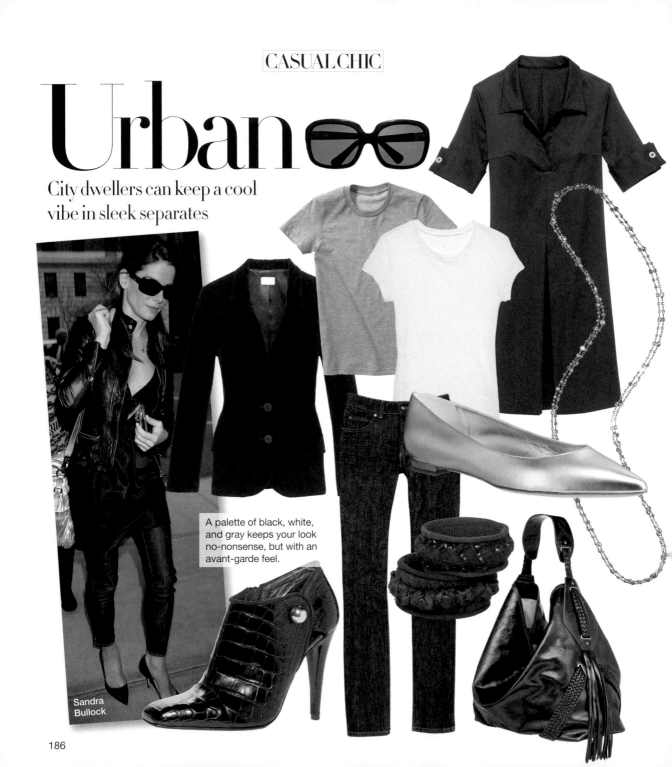

City dwellers can keep a cool vibe in sleek separates

A palette of black, white, and gray keeps your look no-nonsense, but with an avant-garde feel.

Sandra Bullock

186

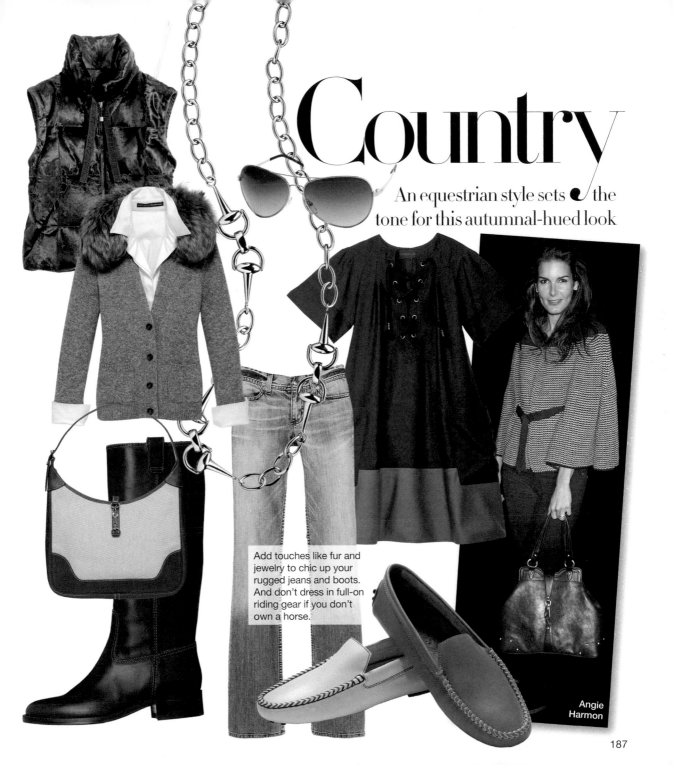

Country

An equestrian style sets the tone for this autumnal-hued look

Add touches like fur and jewelry to chic up your rugged jeans and boots. And don't dress in full-on riding gear if you don't own a horse.

Angie Harmon

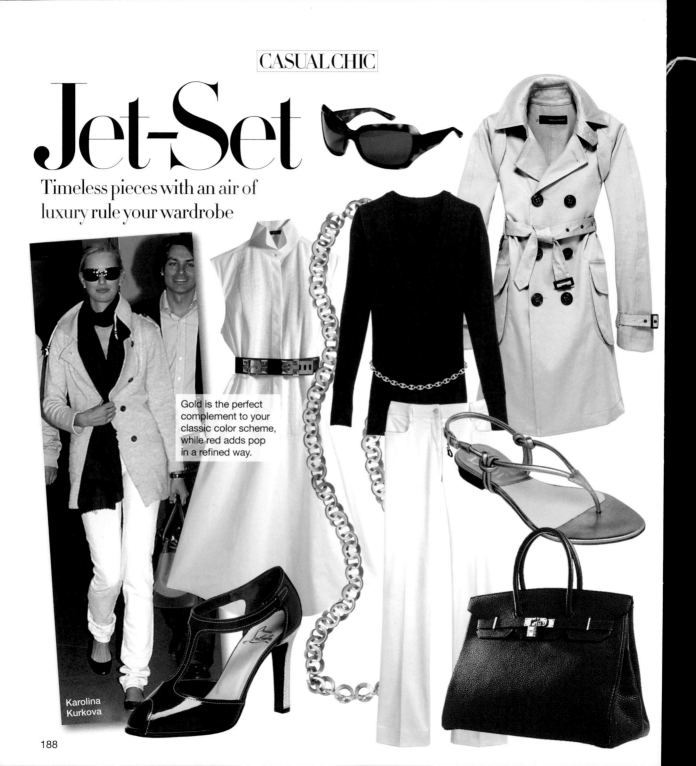

Jet-Set

Timeless pieces with an air of luxury rule your wardrobe

Gold is the perfect complement to your classic color scheme, while red adds pop in a refined way.

Karolina Kurkova

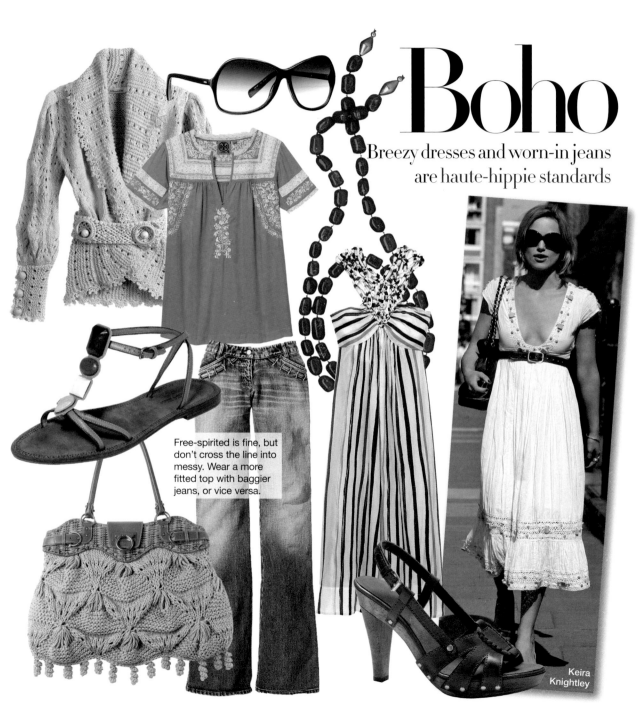

Boho

Breezy dresses and worn-in jeans are haute-hippie standards

Free-spirited is fine, but don't cross the line into messy. Wear a more fitted top with baggier jeans, or vice versa.

Keira Knightley

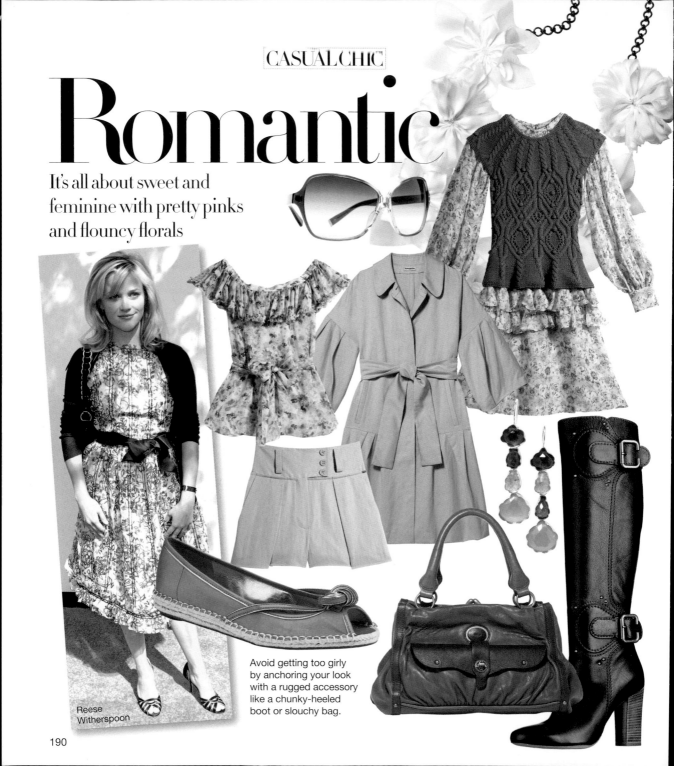

Romantic

It's all about sweet and
feminine with pretty pinks
and flouncy florals

Reese
Witherspoon

Avoid getting too girly
by anchoring your look
with a rugged accessory
like a chunky-heeled
boot or slouchy bag.

190

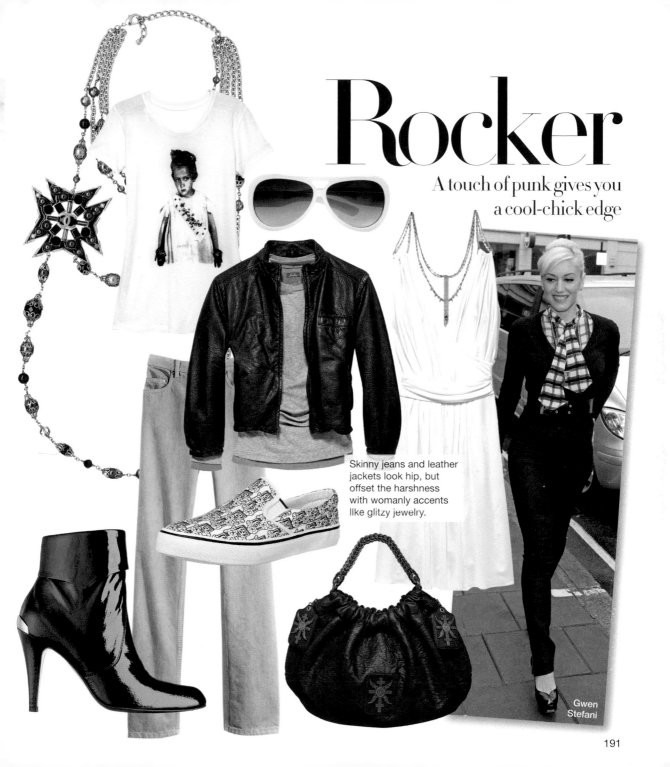

Rocker

A touch of punk gives you a cool-chick edge

Skinny jeans and leather jackets look hip, but offset the harshness with womanly accents like glitzy jewelry.

Gwen Stefani

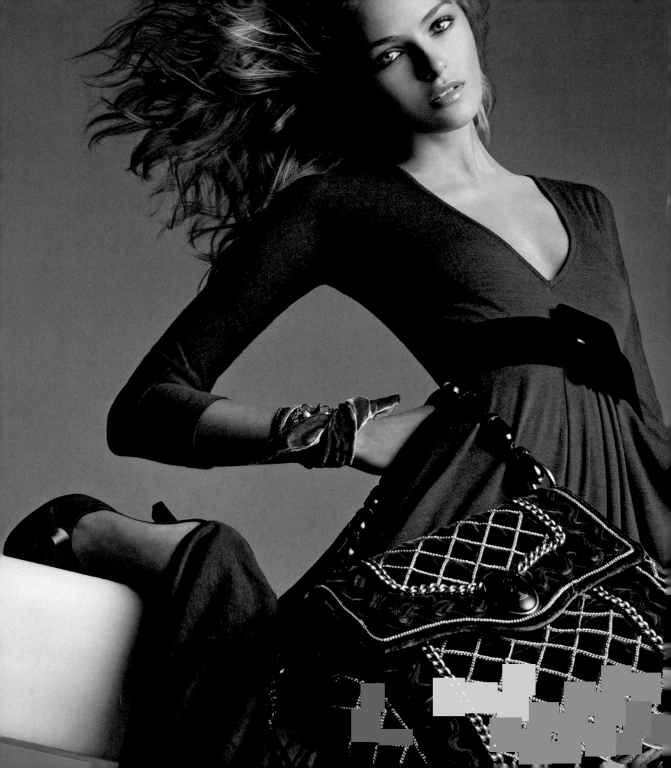

The Best Extras

8. Let accessories complete your look

"You put on high heels and you change."

—MANOLO BLAHNIK

THE BEST EXTRAS

There are reasons so many women, fashion obsessed or not, love—*love, love*—accessories so much. Mostly it's because they have nothing to do with our figure. An amazing shoe, bag, or necklace looks, well, amazing on everyone. But there is something about the sheer joy, the bliss, that purchasing a new tote, pair of high heels, or dangly earrings brings us. It's a euphoric feeling that starts at the moment of purchase and is reexperienced every time you grab that particular piece from the closet. No wonder the word *addict* often follows *accessory*. And the object of our lust could be anything. Bags: big and small. Shoes: flat and tall. Diamonds, beads, bows. Every woman has her own passion when it comes to accents. And it's a passion worth indulging in. Accessories not only finish an outfit, they can set the tone for your look. The switch of a heel to a flat, chandelier earrings to studs, or a slouchy hobo bag to a classic, structured carryall can change the entire effect of the clothes you are wearing. The bottom line is, a girl can't live on clothes alone. Extras are an easy way to add your personality to what you wear.

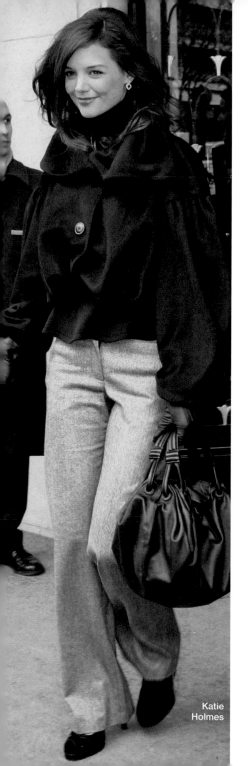

Katie
Holmes

Must-Haves

The 10 necessities of an accessory wardrobe

1. Pumps. Whether they have pointy, round, or square toes, these classic heels look smart at work and sexy at night. Always have a black pair.

2. Flats. Simple ballet slippers or skimmers are a more comfortable answer to the all-purpose pump. They're great for when you're on the go.

3. Diamonds. Rings, earrings, necklaces, bracelets: No matter what form they come in, these sparkly stones will always shine—even if you are wearing jeans and a T-shirt.

4. Pearls. A classic, ladylike staple, these lustrous beads, as tidy little earrings or a single or multistrand necklace, always add polish and elegance to your outfit.

5. A structured bag. In a medium size, a sturdy, top-handle leather bag will serve you well every day.

6. A clutch. For evening, it's essential. A slim, sleek little bag that fits just the necessities is the piece to carry at night.

7. A belt. This piece can turn an ensemble from sloppy to sleek in an instant. It's a good idea to have multiple waist cinchers—thin, medium, and wide—in your closet.

8. A cocktail ring. Give your evening style a glam punch with a big-stoned bauble. Try bold, colorful stones for added effect.

9. A cuff. A thick bracelet in gold, silver, or enamel is a timeless accent and works day or night.

10. A metal watch. A high-quality, classic timepiece like a tank or a bracelet style—whether gold or stainless steel—will last you a lifetime.

> "What woman doesn't love shoes?
> I haven't met one yet." —KATIE HOLMES

Classic Accessories

Some accent pieces have stood the test of time

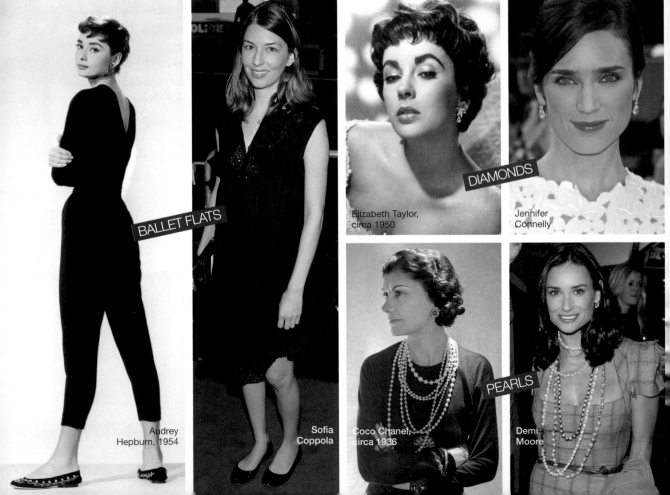

BALLET FLATS

Audrey
Hepburn, 1954

Sofia
Coppola

DIAMONDS

Elizabeth Taylor,
circa 1950

Jennifer
Connelly

PEARLS

Coco Chanel,
circa 1936

Demi
Moore

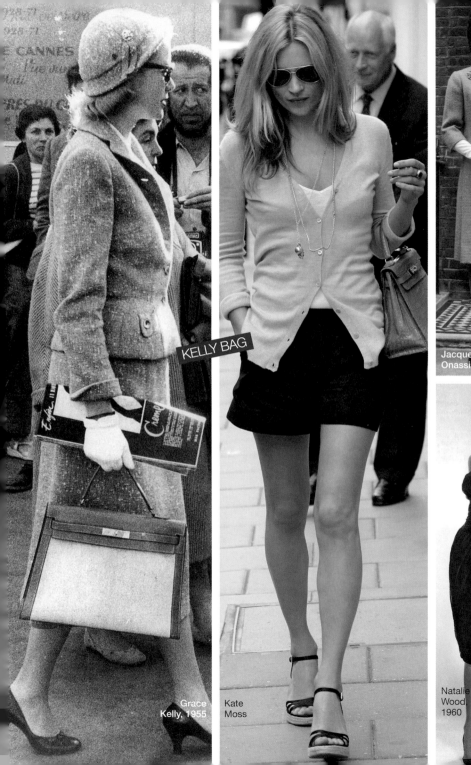

KELLY BAG

Grace
Kelly, 1955

Kate Moss

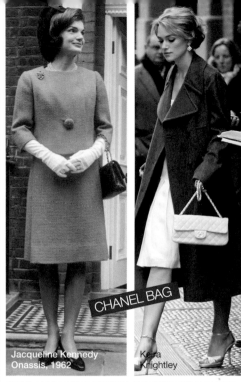

CHANEL BAG

Jacqueline Kennedy
Onassis, 1962

Keira
Knightley

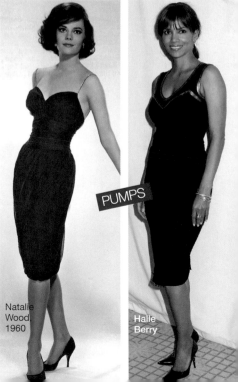

PUMPS

Natalie
Wood,
1960

Halle
Berry

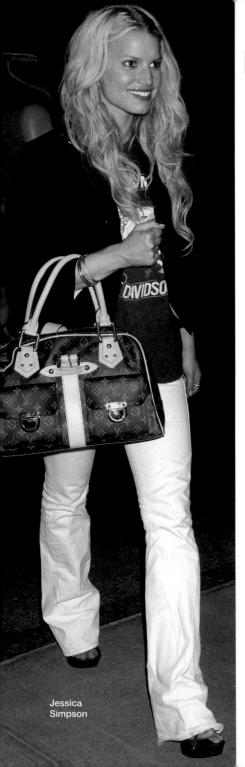

Jessica
Simpson

Bags

The perfect armpiece should be both polished and practical

Most of us can't live without a bag to tote everything we need for the day or night. But just because it's all about function doesn't mean it has to be boring. Special is now standard, so don't feel obligated to buy basics. Have some fun with this necessary accessory.

- **Look for versatility** if you don't have the time, energy, or resources to switch your bag with every outfit. Black and brown go with everything, yes, but so do metallics, skins, and shades of white; they're fresher alternatives.
- **A bright bag adds life to a pared-down look.** Wearing jeans and a tee or a classic dark suit? A carryall in bright orange or pink is an instant pick-me-up.
- **If you find yourself toting a ton, get a larger bag.** A piece that's overstuffed looks sloppy. Doubling up is fine, but don't weigh yourself down. If you have extra items to carry, fill up a large bag to carry along with your regular purse. Better yet, stash your smaller bag in it.
- **Your bag should be relative to your size.** Petite? Don't carry something you could fit in; instead choose something small to medium. Tall and broad? A wee bag will look out of proportion. Try one that's large or oversize.
- **Recognize when it's time to buy a new one,** even if you are attached. Holes, tears, frayed stitching, and worn leather mean your bag needs to be retired.

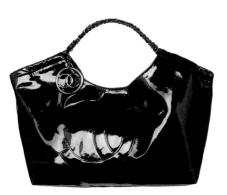

OVERSIZE

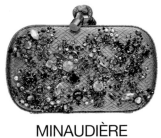

MINAUDIÈRE

CLUTCH

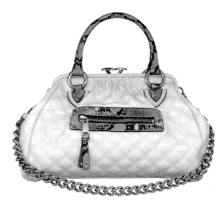

FRAMED

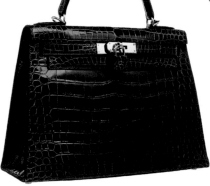

LUXE SKIN

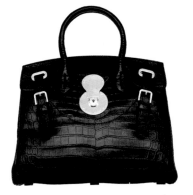

STRUCTURED

"A beautiful, luxurious
handbag conveys glamour
and style to the world."
—DONATELLA VERSACE

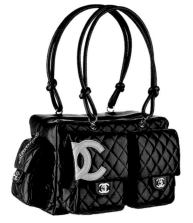

CARGO

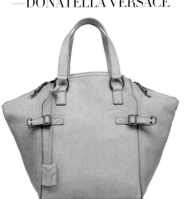

TOTE

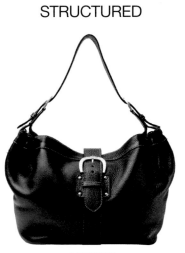

HOBO

Bag Style

Your tote can set the tone for your look

Your accessories are a reflection of your personal aesthetic, so the bag you carry can say a lot about what you are feeling that day or the image you want to project.

- **Soft, slouchy leather says low-key.** Whether it has a hobo shape or cargo pockets, a bag with a worn-in feeling can look rugged but hip. If it's too shabby, though, it's not chic.
- **Top-handle, structured bags are ladylike** and well suited for work and dressier day events.
- **Messenger bags are sporty,** and because you can wear them across your body, they leave your hands free. Look for cuts in canvas and nylon. (Leave the backpacks to school children and hikers.)
- **Add an edge with a studded style.** A bag adorned with heavy metal hardware gives your look a cool vibe.
- **Indulge in sumptuous skins** like ostrich, crocodile, alligator, and python. These luxurious pieces are definitely a splurge, but they're sure to last.

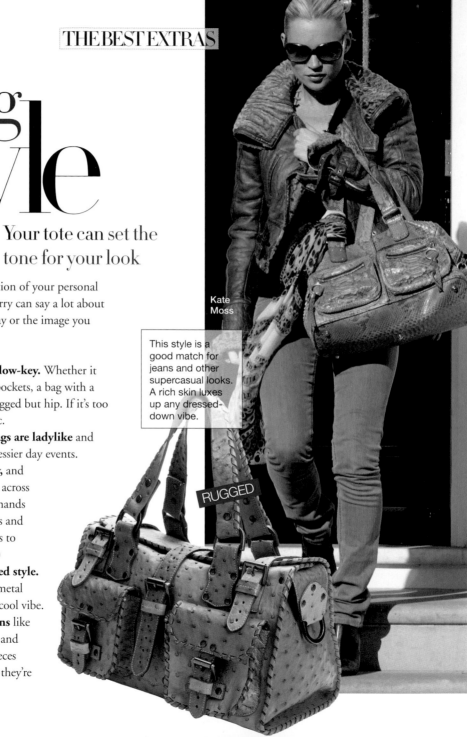

Kate Moss

This style is a good match for jeans and other supercasual looks. A rich skin luxes up any dressed-down vibe.

RUGGED

200

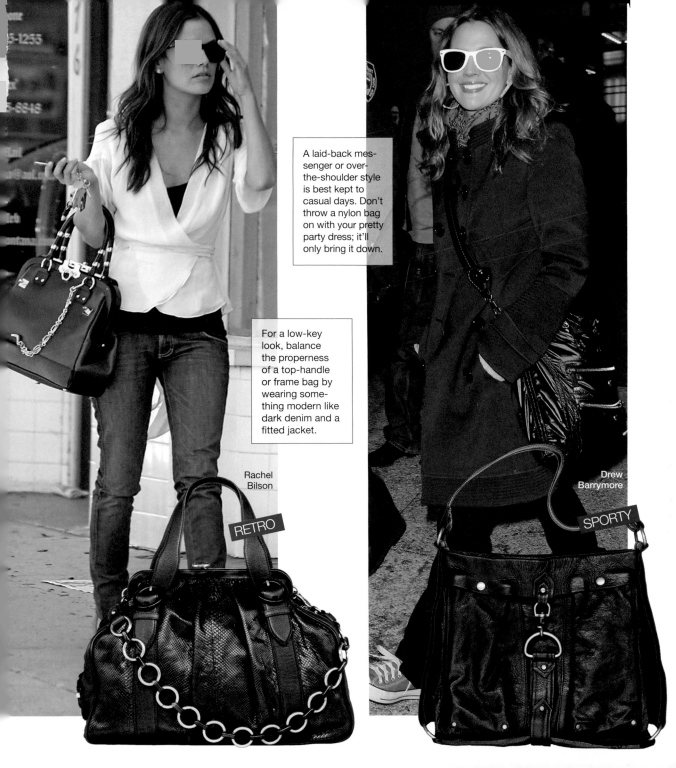

A laid-back messenger or over-the-shoulder style is best kept to casual days. Don't throw a nylon bag on with your pretty party dress; it'll only bring it down.

For a low-key look, balance the properness of a top-handle or frame bag by wearing something modern like dark denim and a fitted jacket.

Rachel Bilson

Drew Barrymore

RETRO

SPORTY

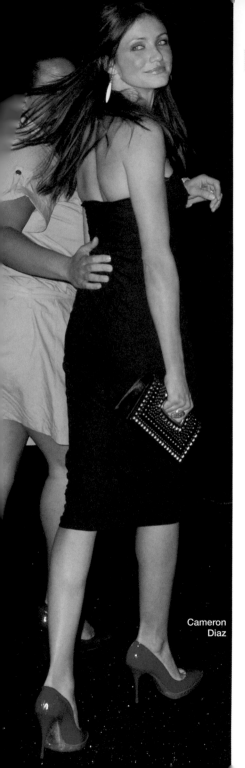

Cameron
Diaz

Shoes

From flats to four-inch heels, you can never have enough footwear

It's no secret that women adore shoes. When you are blue, buying a new pair is an instant mood lifter. When you feel great, you make a trip to the shoe store in celebration. And on special occasions, you *must* have something special to wear. The truth is, there will always be a good excuse to add to your shoe closet.

- **Don't be hobbled by uncomfortable shoes.** Even if you love a pair, if you can't walk in them, don't buy them. Limping around in heels is decidedly ungraceful.
- **Dare to wear brights.** An electric hue can amp up a look, including outfits in colors other than black and denim. Try colored shoes with white, khaki, and pastels. A scarlet-red dress, however, calls for neutral footwear.
- **Let one piece be the attention getter.** If you are wearing an over-the-top dress, for example, keep your shoes toned down. But if your look is low-key, a stand-out shoe adds excitement.
- **Keep in mind what's appropriate.** Open-toe sandals may be too risqué for a conservative suit, while a flat may be too casual for a cocktail frock. Keep your sneakers relegated to gym clothes or casual jeans.
- **For outdoor affairs, spindly stilettos are a no-no.** It will be difficult to walk when your heels keep sinking into the ground, and you'll ruin your shoes. Flats are fine, but if you want height, wedges are an ideal option.

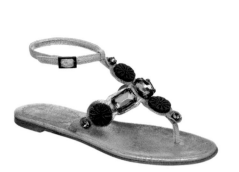

FLAT SANDAL

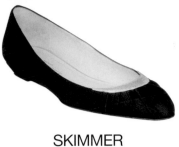

SKIMMER

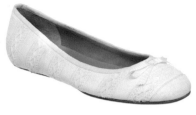

BALLET SLIPPER

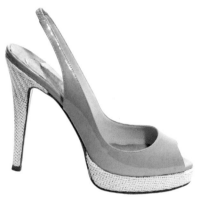

SLINGBACK

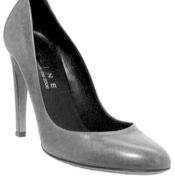

PUMP

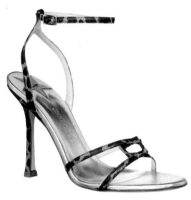

STILETTO

"It is not a quality of putting on high heels to be seductive; a chic woman is born in heels." —MARC JACOBS

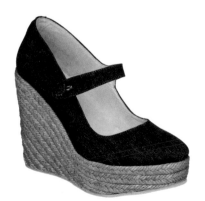

WEDGE

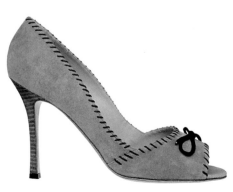

PEEP TOE

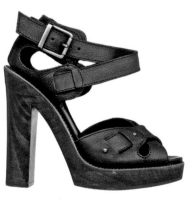

PLATFORM

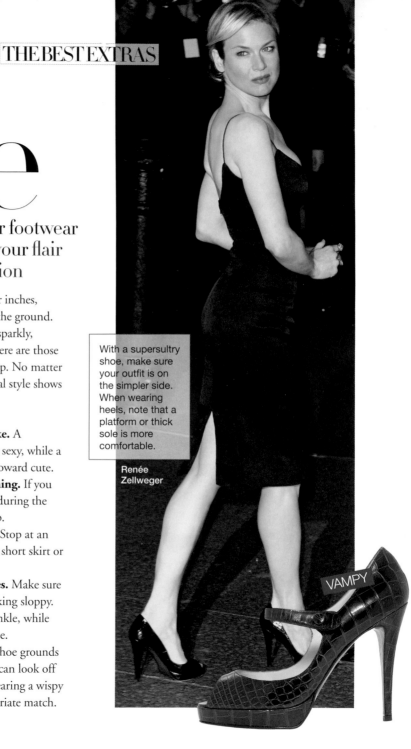

Shoe Style

Let your footwear reflect your flair for fashion

Some of us won't wear heels less than four inches, while others insist on remaining close to the ground. Many of us have a closet filled with only sparkly, sequined, and metallic shoes, and then there are those who have 20 pairs of the same black pump. No matter which category you fall into, your personal style shows in your shoes.

- **Know what statement you want to make.** A spindly stiletto sandal is all about looking sexy, while a bow-emblazoned kitten heel veers more toward cute.
- **Va-va-voom shoes have their place: evening.** If you still want to wear a knock-'em-dead look during the day, choose a closed-toe or peep-toe pump.
- **Sky-high shoes call for tame hemlines.** Stop at an inch above the knee. But when wearing a short skirt or dress, wear a lower heel or flat.
- **Pair flats with properly hemmed clothes.** Make sure your clothing is tailored or you'll risk looking sloppy. A trouser leg should fall at or above the ankle, while skirts or dresses should end above the knee.
- **Think about balance.** A thicker-heeled shoe grounds a heavily layered look. Something dainty can look off balance. The reverse holds true. When wearing a wispy frock, a thin-strapped sandal is an appropriate match.

With a supersultry shoe, make sure your outfit is on the simpler side. When wearing heels, note that a platform or thick sole is more comfortable.

Renée Zellweger

VAMPY

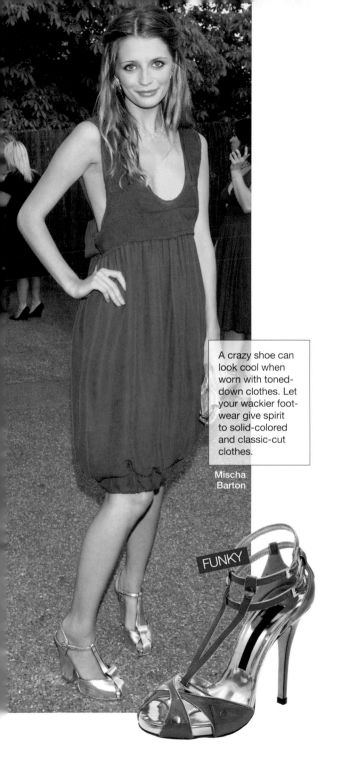

A crazy shoe can look cool when worn with toned-down clothes. Let your wackier footwear give spirit to solid-colored and classic-cut clothes.

Mischa Barton

FUNKY

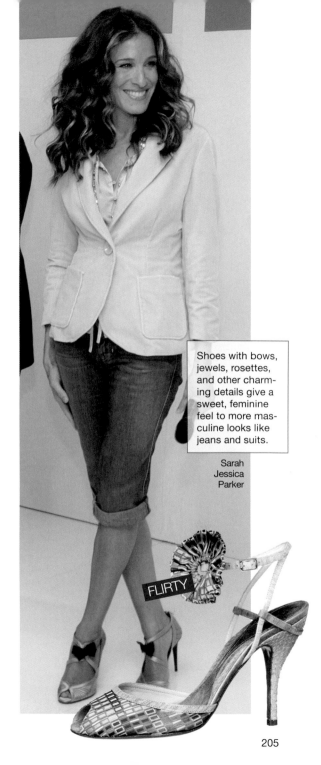

Shoes with bows, jewels, rosettes, and other charming details give a sweet, feminine feel to more masculine looks like jeans and suits.

Sarah Jessica Parker

FLIRTY

205

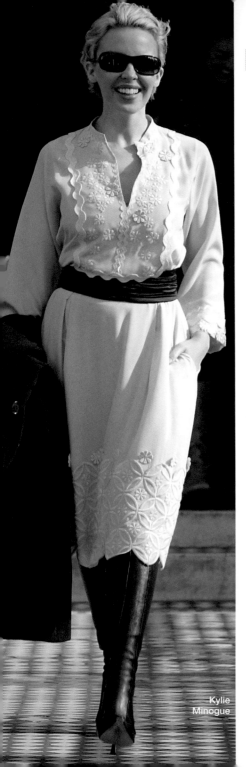

Kylie
Minogue

Boots

Whether classic or edgy, this full-coverage footwear can be comfortable *and* chic

Why do we love boots so much? They can have a rugged country look, an equestrian vibe, or a sleek urban air. On chillier days, they make dresses and skirts wearable. They also give polish to jeans and add a down-to-earth feel to more delicate pieces. Boots increase the versatility of your clothes, and every woman should have a pair or two.

- **High boots keep you warm** and are perfect for fall and winter days. They allow you to get wear out of your lighter dresses and skirts when it's cold. Put them in the back of your closet when the temperatures start to rise, though; they look out of place in hot weather.
- **A high-heel boot can be just as ladylike as a pump.** When wearing a fuller skirt, it's more refined for your hem to fall just over the top of your boot. With a fitted shape, allow a few inches between your hem and your boot.
- **Short skirts look tarty with stiletto, thigh-high boots.** Wear a flat style with a mini. Think about wearing tights, too; you'll look more conservative and pulled together.
- **Heavier-heeled styles complement longer skirts** and dresses. But don't put a beat-up boot with your tiered skirt. Save your rough-and-tumble footwear for jeans.
- **Ankle boots are a wonderful option.** They slip easily under pants and don't feel restrictive around your legs.

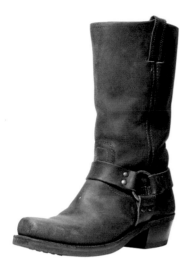

RUGGED

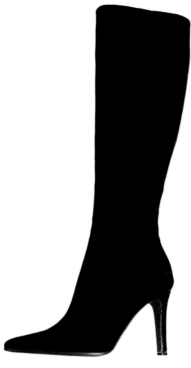

HIGH HEEL

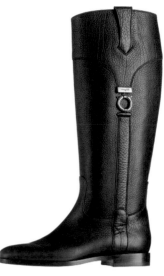

RIDING

"Accessories are the face-lift of tired or older clothes."
—KARL LAGERFELD

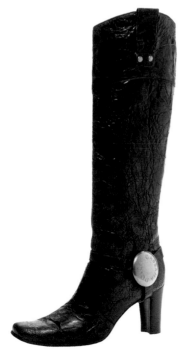

MILITARY

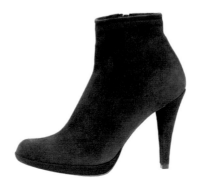

ANKLE BOOT

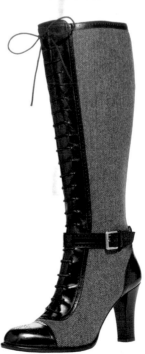

LACE-UP

Boot Style

The right pair can transform your look

Make no mistake about it, you can expect boots to be a prominent part of your ensemble, so choose what you wear wisely. But once you have a pair you like, you'll get lots of use out of them. They may be more expensive than shoes, but they're worth it.

- **A slim, high boot is a staple.** Pick a pair that's fitted around your leg but not so tight that your skin bulges out from the top. There shouldn't be more than a half inch of space between your leg and your boot.
- **Flat equestrian-style boots can be less fitted.** A straight cut makes them easy to slip in and out of, and they're perfect if you want to put your jeans inside. They're a little more casual but still refined.
- **Leather boots ground flowy frocks,** giving them a down-to-earth feel.
- **Tuck your slim jeans into slim, high-heel boots** for a glamorous air, but this really works best only on the skinny minnies among us.
- **Soft, slouchy boots have a '70s vibe** and work well with skinny pants or longer skirts.
- **For an ultramodern edge, try ankle boots,** or booties.

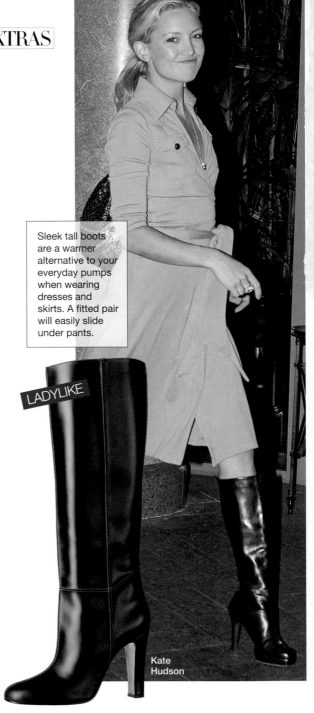

Sleek tall boots are a warmer alternative to your everyday pumps when wearing dresses and skirts. A fitted pair will easily slide under pants.

LADYLIKE

Kate Hudson

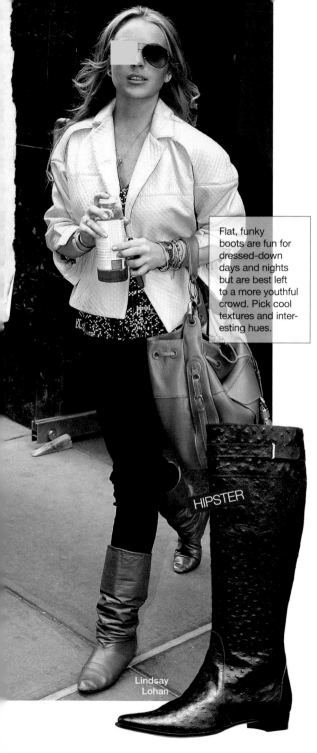

Flat, funky boots are fun for dressed-down days and nights but are best left to a more youthful crowd. Pick cool textures and interesting hues.

HIPSTER

Lindsay Lohan

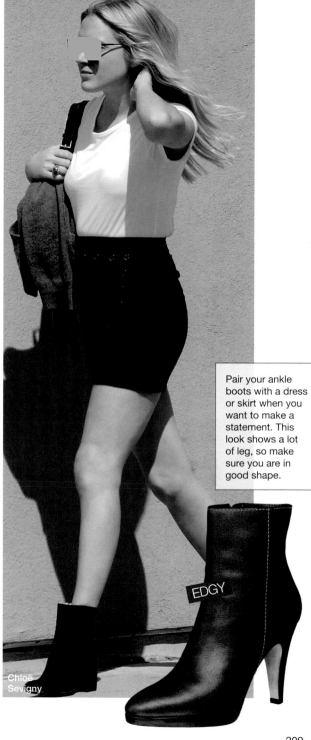

Pair your ankle boots with a dress or skirt when you want to make a statement. This look shows a lot of leg, so make sure you are in good shape.

EDGY

Chloë Sevigny

209

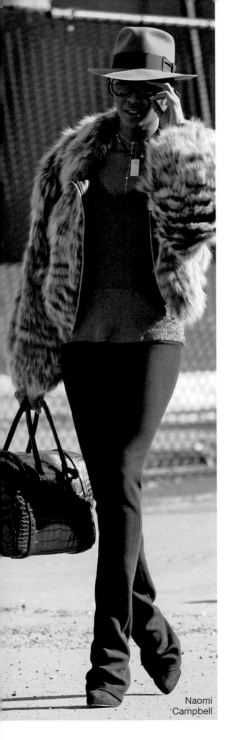

Naomi
Campbell

Perfect

Some pieces look better worn together

Pairings

We've come a long way from the days of matchy-matchy shoes and bags, when women actually bought the two as a set. Now we can be a lot more creative when deciding what goes with what.

- **Combine textures.** A patent boot with a patent tote is way too much patent. But a high-gloss shoe with a plush velvet bag (or vice versa) offers just the right amount of shine.
- **Put prints with solids.** Don't double up on a loud pattern; balance busy with basic. But that doesn't mean you should shy away from color. Leopard print looks incredibly chic paired with bright red.
- **Mix metallic and matte.** Shimmery silver looks sleek with black, while bronze or gold is a good buddy for brown.
- **Stay in one style.** Your earthy equestrian boots call for an equally earthy hobo bag. Grab a sleek clutch when teetering in your sexy stilettos, a dainty purse with your ladylike pumps, a sporty nylon messenger bag with your sneaks, and so on.

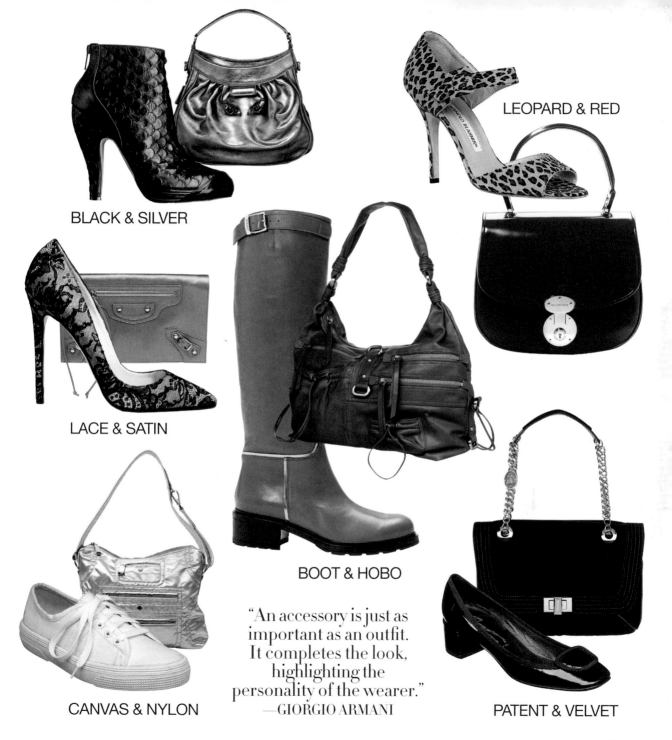

BLACK & SILVER

LEOPARD & RED

LACE & SATIN

BOOT & HOBO

CANVAS & NYLON

"An accessory is just as important as an outfit. It completes the look, highlighting the personality of the wearer."
—GIORGIO ARMANI

PATENT & VELVET

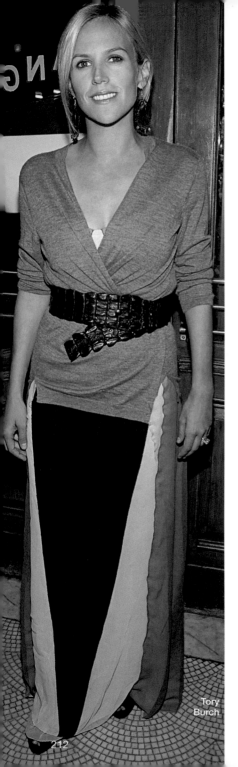

Tory
Burch

Belts

Look clean-cut by cinching your waist

It's amazing how a simple belt can totally modify an outfit. With the quick closing of a buckle, almost anything you wear is instantly pulled together, and you suddenly look slimmer. And we're not just talking about the basic leather piece used to hold up pants. If a wide-cut piece like a sash or obi emphasizes your waist, it'll do the trick.

- **Look at belts in a new light.** When worn out of the belt loops of your pants, they can go over nearly everything. Cinch a bulky sweater, a slouchy tee, or a billowing blouse. Even try it over your coat for a more tailored look.
- **They should flatter your figure.** Wearing your belt on your true waist (as opposed to the top of your pants) will create a feminine hourglass silhouette. A low-slung belt over jeans or a dress can be cool and casual.
- **Get in on a new trend subtly with a belt.** Pick a piece in the color or print du jour and get a touch of the latest style without buying a whole new outfit.
- **A belt can act like jewelry.** A loose chain that hangs low can add a touch of glitz in an understated way. Don't pile on the necklaces when going this route.

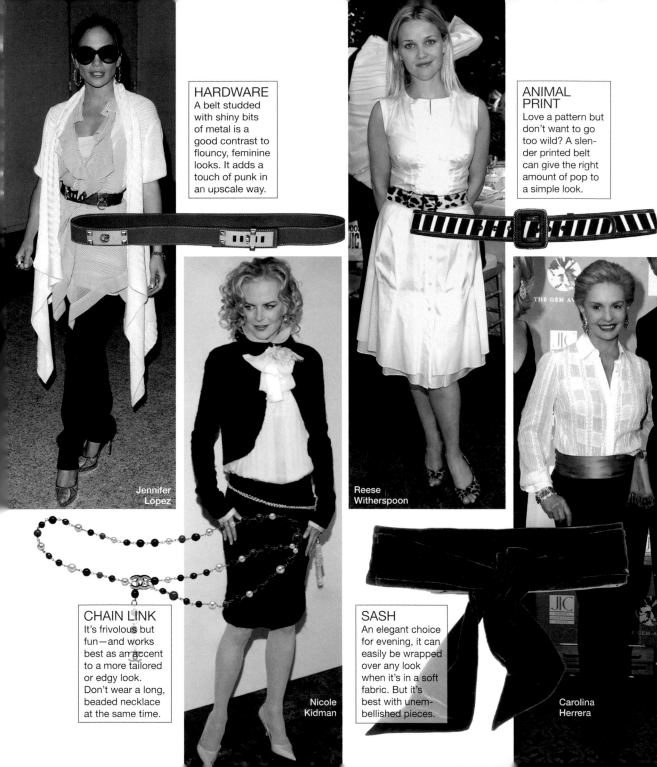

HARDWARE
A belt studded with shiny bits of metal is a good contrast to flouncy, feminine looks. It adds a touch of punk in an upscale way.

ANIMAL PRINT
Love a pattern but don't want to go too wild? A slender printed belt can give the right amount of pop to a simple look.

Jennifer Lopez

Reese Witherspoon

CHAIN LINK
It's frivolous but fun—and works best as an accent to a more tailored or edgy look. Don't wear a long, beaded necklace at the same time.

Nicole Kidman

SASH
An elegant choice for evening, it can easily be wrapped over any look when it's in a soft fabric. But it's best with unembellished pieces.

Carolina Herrera

Jewelry

Whether fancy or costume, a bit of bling is never a bad thing

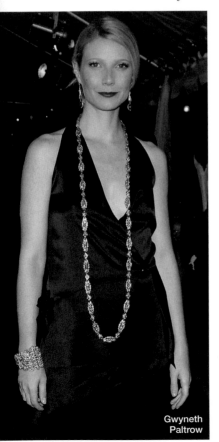

Gwyneth
Paltrow

There is nothing that brings a smile to our face like a pretty ring, a jangly necklace, or some sparkly earrings. Big or small, real or fake, understated or over-the-top, jewelry lifts the spirits. It also lifts a look. Colorful beads or chandelier earrings could be just the thing to make an ordinary outfit outstanding. While jewelry is a very personal thing—gifts from your significant other, family heirlooms, purchases to mark milestones—it can also be a reflection of your style spirit. Some people can't go out of the house without loading up necklaces, while for others simple studs will do. Some women prefer an armful of bangles, and some load up on brooches. No matter your preference, bits of baubles are all about adding joy to your look.

- **Keep it chic.** In some instances, loading up on the sparklies is an exciting way to accent. But know when to stop. An armful of bangles, for example, means you should think minimal with your necklaces and earrings.
- **Tone it down when your clothes** have a lot going on. A ruffle-front blouse can look sweet with a thin chain in the mix, but not with a big, ornate number.
- **You don't have to spend a lot on your baubles.** Costume jewelry adds pizzazz. Beware of anything too cheap, and avoid pieces that are just poor imitations of the real deal.

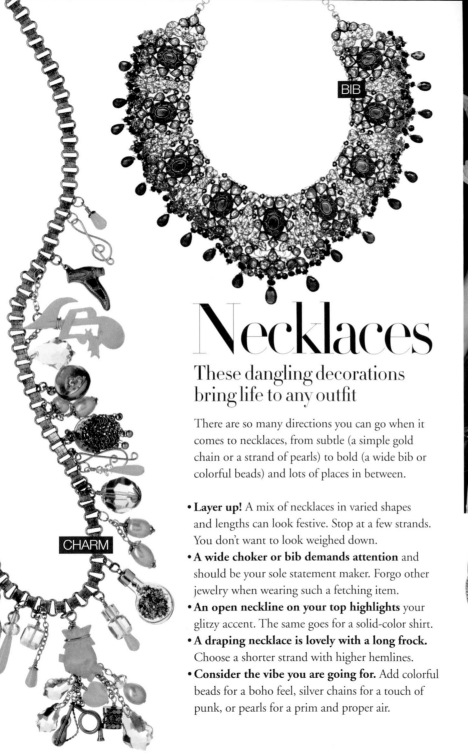
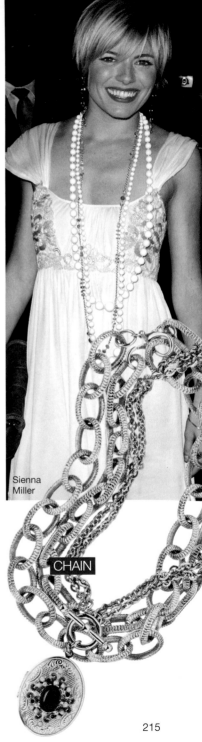

BIB

CHARM

CHAIN

Sienna Miller

Necklaces

These dangling decorations bring life to any outfit

There are so many directions you can go when it comes to necklaces, from subtle (a simple gold chain or a strand of pearls) to bold (a wide bib or colorful beads) and lots of places in between.

- **Layer up!** A mix of necklaces in varied shapes and lengths can look festive. Stop at a few strands. You don't want to look weighed down.
- **A wide choker or bib demands attention** and should be your sole statement maker. Forgo other jewelry when wearing such a fetching item.
- **An open neckline on your top highlights** your glitzy accent. The same goes for a solid-color shirt.
- **A draping necklace is lovely with a long frock.** Choose a shorter strand with higher hemlines.
- **Consider the vibe you are going for.** Add colorful beads for a boho feel, silver chains for a touch of punk, or pearls for a prim and proper air.

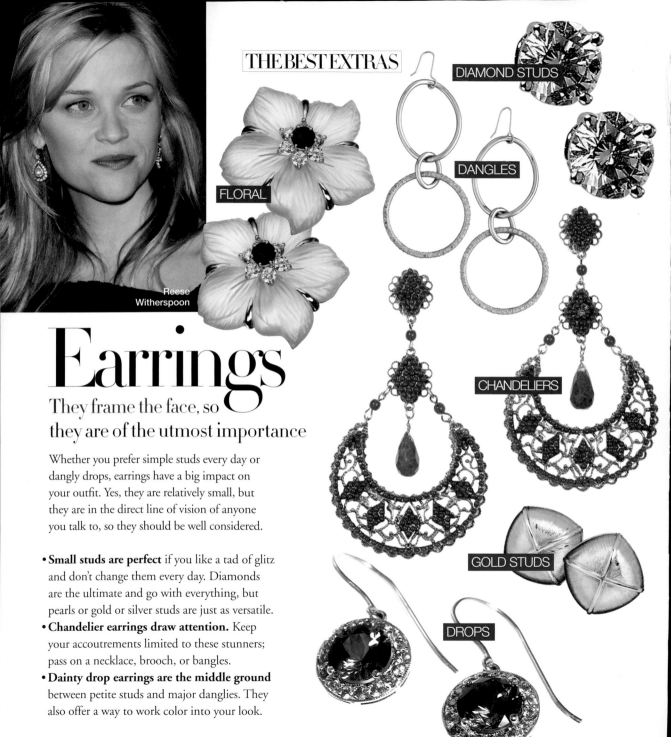

DIAMOND STUDS

FLORAL

DANGLES

CHANDELIERS

Reese
Witherspoon

Earrings

They frame the face, so they are of the utmost importance

Whether you prefer simple studs every day or dangly drops, earrings have a big impact on your outfit. Yes, they are relatively small, but they are in the direct line of vision of anyone you talk to, so they should be well considered.

- **Small studs are perfect** if you like a tad of glitz and don't change them every day. Diamonds are the ultimate and go with everything, but pearls or gold or silver studs are just as versatile.
- **Chandelier earrings draw attention.** Keep your accoutrements limited to these stunners; pass on a necklace, brooch, or bangles.
- **Dainty drop earrings are the middle ground** between petite studs and major danglies. They also offer a way to work color into your look.

GOLD STUDS

DROPS

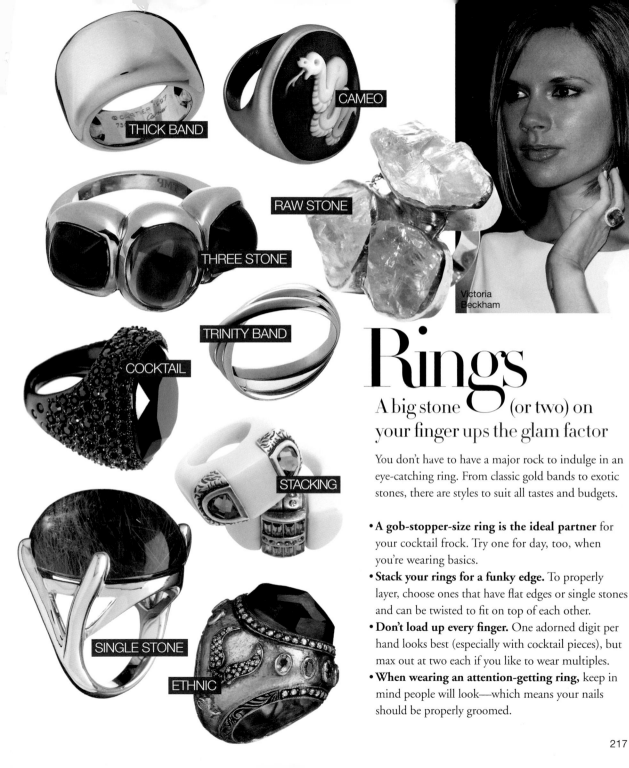

THICK BAND

CAMEO

RAW STONE

THREE STONE

Victoria Beckham

TRINITY BAND

COCKTAIL

STACKING

SINGLE STONE

ETHNIC

Rings

A big stone (or two) on your finger ups the glam factor

You don't have to have a major rock to indulge in an eye-catching ring. From classic gold bands to exotic stones, there are styles to suit all tastes and budgets.

- **A gob-stopper-size ring is the ideal partner** for your cocktail frock. Try one for day, too, when you're wearing basics.
- **Stack your rings for a funky edge.** To properly layer, choose ones that have flat edges or single stones and can be twisted to fit on top of each other.
- **Don't load up every finger.** One adorned digit per hand looks best (especially with cocktail pieces), but max out at two each if you like to wear multiples.
- **When wearing an attention-getting ring,** keep in mind people will look—which means your nails should be properly groomed.

217

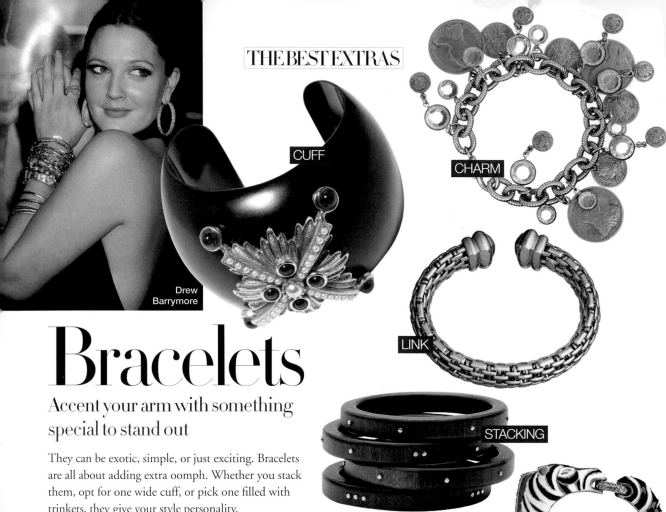

CUFF

CHARM

Drew
Barrymore

LINK

Bracelets

Accent your arm with something special to stand out

They can be exotic, simple, or just exciting. Bracelets are all about adding extra oomph. Whether you stack them, opt for one wide cuff, or pick one filled with trinkets, they give your style personality.

- **Try loading up on an armful.** Stacked bangles—especially gold pieces of varying sizes—put a worldly spin on your style. Add a watch into the mix. Don't go so far that you are jangling everywhere you go.
- **Mixing material can look rich** when wearing multiple bracelets, but keep it limited to one or two types.
- **Lots of bracelets calls for bare wrists.** Wear short sleeves or roll up long ones to display your bijoux.
- **One wide cuff makes an impression.** So, leave the rest of your look toned down. Cuffs can easily slide over a long-sleeved knit. It's a chic way to wear them.

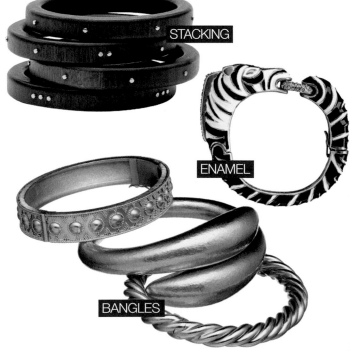

STACKING

ENAMEL

BANGLES

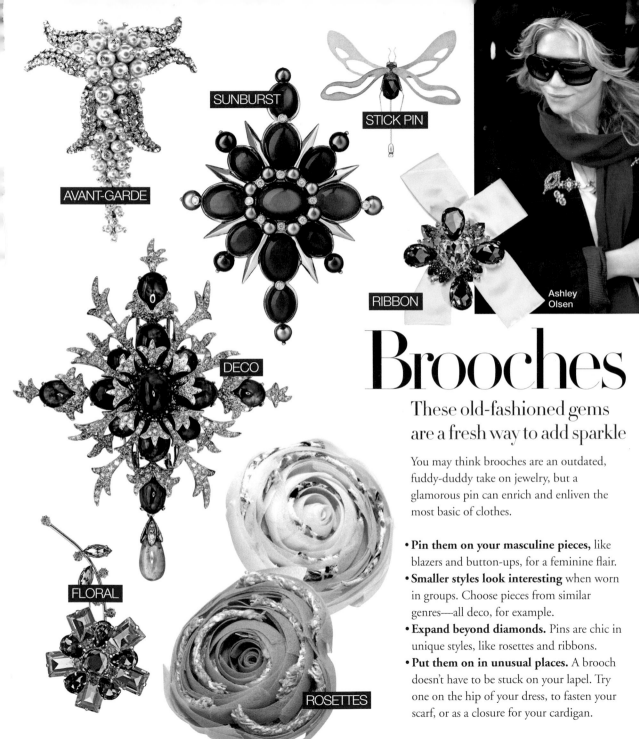

AVANT-GARDE

SUNBURST

STICK PIN

RIBBON

Ashley
Olsen

DECO

FLORAL

ROSETTES

Brooches

These old-fashioned gems are a fresh way to add sparkle

You may think brooches are an outdated, fuddy-duddy take on jewelry, but a glamorous pin can enrich and enliven the most basic of clothes.

- **Pin them on your masculine pieces,** like blazers and button-ups, for a feminine flair.
- **Smaller styles look interesting** when worn in groups. Choose pieces from similar genres—all deco, for example.
- **Expand beyond diamonds.** Pins are chic in unique styles, like rosettes and ribbons.
- **Put them on in unusual places.** A brooch doesn't have to be stuck on your lapel. Try one on the hip of your dress, to fasten your scarf, or as a closure for your cardigan.

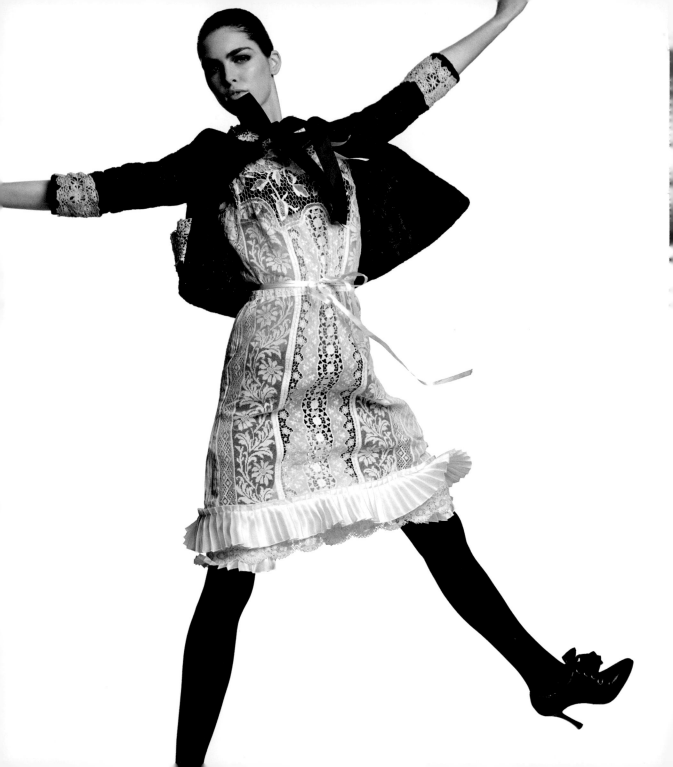

Lingerie Essentials

9. Look good under your clothes

"The greatest concubines in history knew that everything revealed with **nothing concealed** is a bore."
— GEOFFREY BEENE

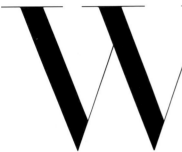

We all fantasize about being one of those women who have devastatingly sultry (and matching) bras and underwear from some exclusive Parisian boutique hidden under their cardigan and pencil skirt. But, alas, we've been lazily content with our old standbys and outdated pieces that could use some refreshing. In fact, most of us, whether we want to admit it or not, are wearing the wrong size bra—85 percent of American women, to be exact. The worst part about having your lingerie drawer filled with ill-fitting, supportless unmentionables is that it limits what you can wear. There is no reason you have to pass on a dress you covet, or even a simple tee, because you don't have the right bra to wear underneath. There are plenty of pieces out there to suit the needs of all women. We don't have to indulge in only the sexiest pieces (although that would be nice); a few good basics will do. The lacy, ruffly numbers are just icing on the cake.

The Perfect Fit

How to determine the right bra size

1. Your bra should fit firmly and evenly around the rib cage and shouldn't ride up in the back. The shoulder straps should be snug without digging in. The larger you are, the wider your straps should be. Also, put your bra on while bending over at the waist, and make sure the cups are filled but not brimming over.

2. Use the middle hook on the back strap. That way, if the bra stretches out or shrinks a touch (or you do), you can tighten it or loosen it to whatever is most comfortable.

3. Try on several sizes for each style, as they may vary by brand and shape. If you are a 32B in one bra, you may be a 34A in another.

4. Seek help. In most lingerie stores, salespeople will happily measure you and help determine the best styles for you.

5. Maximize the life span of your intimates by hand washing them in cold water with gentle detergent. If you must use the washing machine, hook the bra and put it in a net bag.

> "It's important to feel good about your body, and lingerie is a great way of being in touch with it." —ELLE MACPHERSON

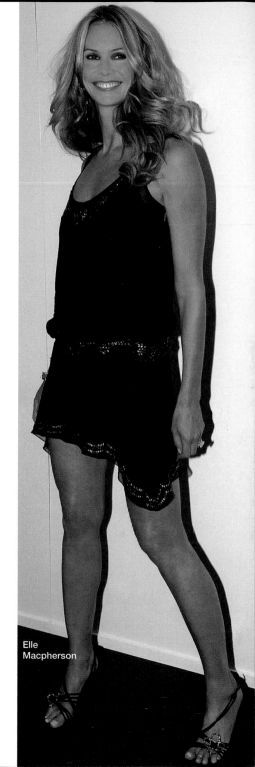

Elle Macpherson

Foundation
Fundamentals

The pieces to have in your lingerie drawer

1. A nude bra. Wear it under your white and light-hued clothing. It should be seamless and slightly padded.

2. A black bra. Wear it under darks, for day or night. Don't put them under light colors.

3. A strapless bra. This is essential for evening and under anything with thin straps or a halter neck.

4. A T-back bra. Use it with tank tops and pieces that cut in at the shoulders and back. Have nude on hand for white tanks or black for black.

5. A convertible bra. It's a sensible purchase that can easily switch from regular to strapless to T-back.

6. A bra for a plunging neckline. Wear it under tops and dresses with deep V-necks. It will get a lot of use at night, so black is a good choice.

7. A supersexy bra and panty. Something frivolous and oh so seductive is worth it, even if you wear it only once.

8. Two sports bras. Stock up on more if you exercise regularly—and replace often, as they wear out fast.

9. Three pairs of underwear for each bra. Whether you prefer thongs or styles with full coverage, it makes sense to have some of each.

10. Three extra fancy pairs of underwear. Every woman should indulge in a few pieces of risqué, playful, or sultry panties just for fun.

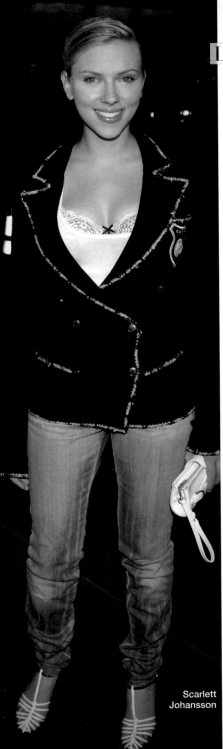

Scarlett
Johansson

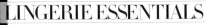

Best Basics

Your undergarments deserve consideration, too

Big or small, we all need a little support, yet the practical pieces we wear every day often get less of our attention than their sexy siblings due to the fact that they are all about function. Because our basic bras and underwear actually get the most use, we should give them a little more thought.

- **Assess your lingerie drawer every year.** Keep in mind that a good bra lasts two to five years, depending how well you've cared for it. (Wear it no more than twice before washing.) You should get refitted for bras when your body goes through a major change like pregnancy.
- **When you find lingerie you love,** that fits well, and that you end up wearing all the time, buy in multiples.
- **If your shirt allows for a touch of bra to show,** wear one that's trimmed in lace or has a little bow detail. A plain basic peeking out is not attractive.
- **When it comes to matching** your bra with your underwear, there are no rules. You are the only one who knows what you've got on under your clothes. If you buy both at one time—and purchase multiple panties for every bra—you'll be able to match without putting much effort into it.
- **Boy shorts are cozy to sleep in** but rarely fit smoothly under clothes, except maybe voluminous skirts.

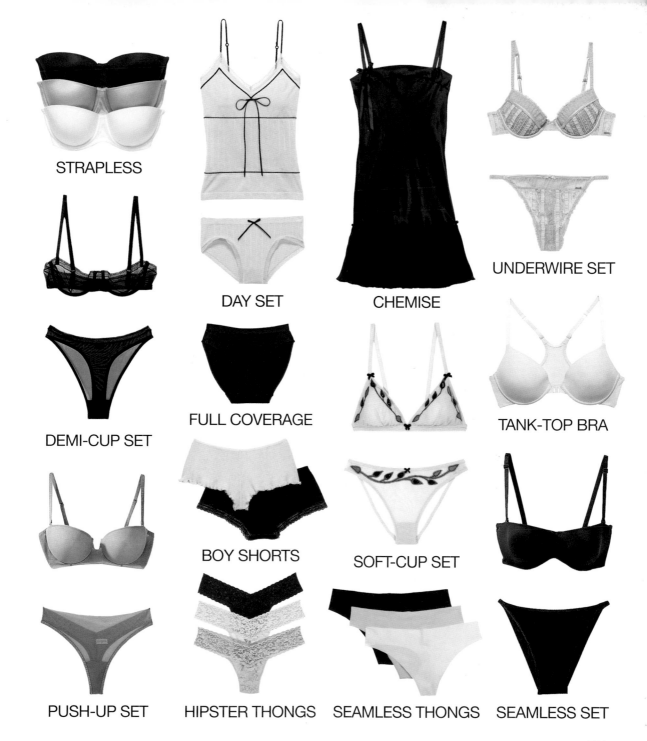

STRAPLESS

DAY SET

CHEMISE

UNDERWIRE SET

DEMI-CUP SET

FULL COVERAGE

TANK-TOP BRA

PUSH-UP SET

BOY SHORTS

SOFT-CUP SET

HIPSTER THONGS

SEAMLESS THONGS

SEAMLESS SET

227

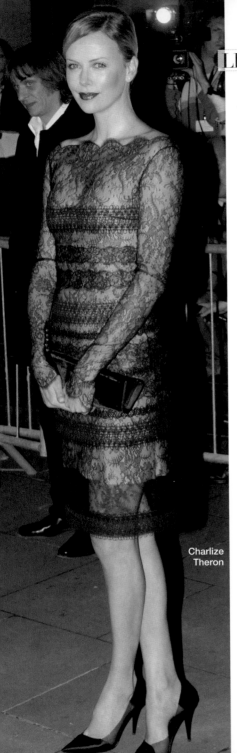

Charlize
Theron

Sexy Staples

We all should indulge in a few lacy, frilly, teeny numbers

Once you get your basics down, it's time to have a little fun with your lingerie. Of course, your significant other will no doubt appreciate it if you spice up your undergarments. More important, wearing something beautiful under your clothes will make you feel good. Whether your style is sheer and slinky, flirty and full of frills, or even fetishy, you should have part of your lingerie wardrobe devoted to these intimates.

- **It's okay to let a little lingerie show at night,** but keep it clean. Lace peeking out of your blouse or dress can be sexy; showing your entire bra is not.
- **Camisoles can be worn out of the bedroom,** under a sweater or on their own. But you should always be properly supported. The same goes for chemises: Wear them as slipdresses, but don't go sans undergarments when wearing them out of the house.
- **Don't wear black lacy pieces under a white T-shirt** or button-up. It looks trashy.
- **If you have a fancy set you want to wear out** at night but your ruffly matching underwear doesn't lie smoothly under your fitted dress or skirt, swap it for a thin black thong. It won't detract from the allure.

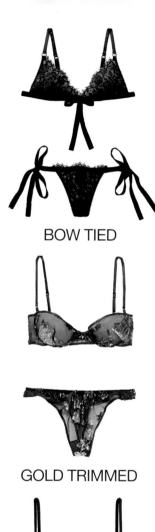

BOW TIED

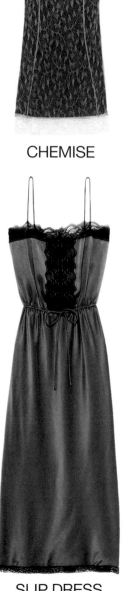

CHEMISE

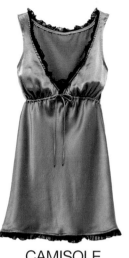

CAMISOLE

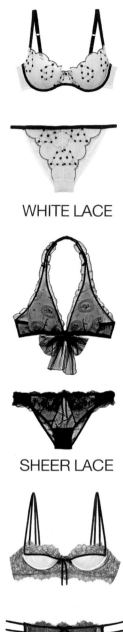

WHITE LACE

GOLD TRIMMED

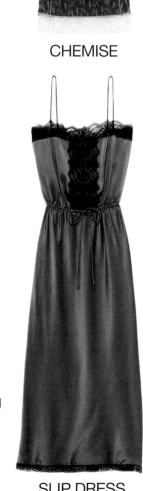

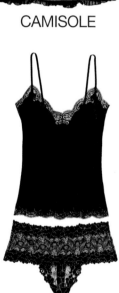

EVENING SET

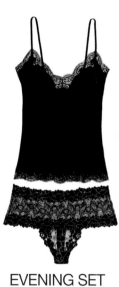

SHEER LACE

PUSH-UP SET

SLIP DRESS

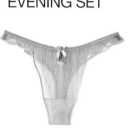

SHEER THONG

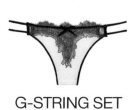

G-STRING SET

229

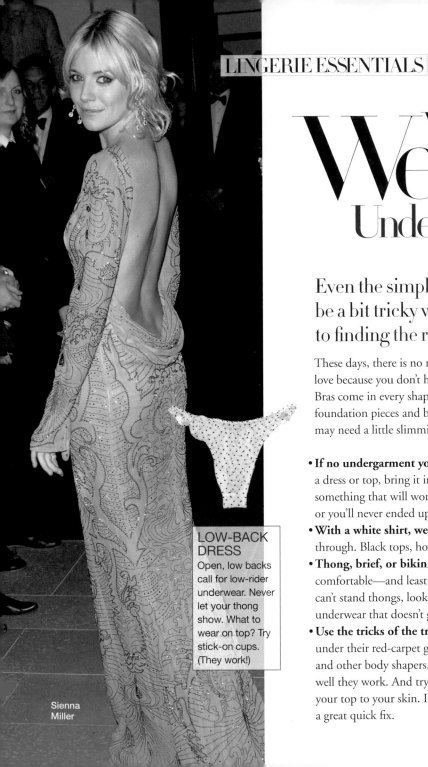

Sienna Miller

What to Wear Under Your...

Even the simplest pieces can be a bit tricky when it comes to finding the right support

These days, there is no reason to sacrifice a look you love because you don't have the right undergarments. Bras come in every shape imaginable. There are foundation pieces and body shapers for any area that may need a little slimming or padding up.

- **If no undergarment you own seems to work** under a dress or top, bring it into the lingerie shop to find something that will work. Take care of it right away or you'll never ended up wearing that difficult piece.
- **With a white shirt, wear a nude bra.** White shows through. Black tops, however, call for black bras.
- **Thong, brief, or bikini?** Whatever is most comfortable—and least noticeable. For those who can't stand thongs, look for full-coverage seamless underwear that doesn't give you visible panty lines.
- **Use the tricks of the trade.** What do the stars wear under their red-carpet gowns? Spandex, control top, and other body shapers. You'd be surprised at how well they work. And try double-stick tape to adhere your top to your skin. If it isn't lying just right, this is a great quick fix.

LOW-BACK DRESS
Open, low backs call for low-rider underwear. Never let your thong show. What to wear on top? Try stick-on cups. (They work!)

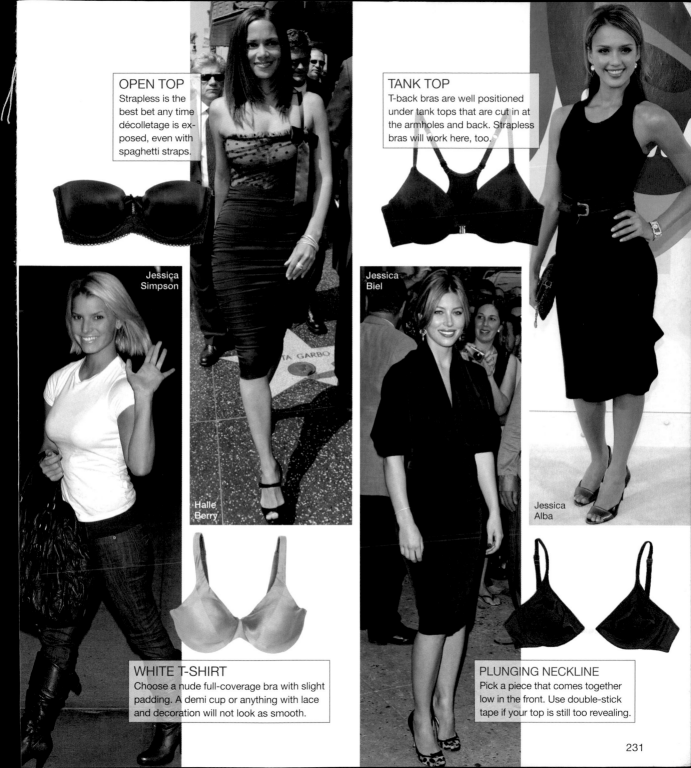

OPEN TOP
Strapless is the best bet any time décolletage is exposed, even with spaghetti straps.

TANK TOP
T-back bras are well positioned under tank tops that are cut in at the armholes and back. Strapless bras will work here, too.

Jessica Simpson

Halle Berry

Jessica Biel

Jessica Alba

WHITE T-SHIRT
Choose a nude full-coverage bra with slight padding. A demi cup or anything with lace and decoration will not look as smooth.

PLUNGING NECKLINE
Pick a piece that comes together low in the front. Use double-stick tape if your top is still too revealing.

The 10 Commandments of Dressing

When contemplating a purchase or just deciding what to wear, consider these tenets and you can't go wrong

1. Know what you like and what you don't.

2. Dress for yourself—not for anyone else.

3. Dress to suit your age.

4. Dress to suit your shape.

5. Look appropriate for where you are going.

6. Wear your clothes with confidence.

7. Feel good about what you spend your money on.

8. Embrace your individual style.

9. Don't be a slave to the latest trend.

10. Don't be afraid to break the rules.

Index

Accessories, 193–219. *See also* Bags;
  Jewelry; Shoes
    accenting LBD, 135
    belts, 123, 195, 212–213
    classics, 196–197
    enhancing eveningwear, 139,
      143, 147, 153
    freshening up office basics,
      122–123
    for less conservative suits,
      116–121
    for metallics and sequins, 143
    must-haves, 195
    for night brights, 139
    from office to cocktails, 152–153
    overview, 194–195
    for tuxedos, 147
Age-specific advice, 51–77
    20s, 53, 54–57, 116
    30s, 53, 58–61, 117
    40s, 53, 62–65, 118
    50s, 53, 66–69, 119
    60s, 53, 70–73, 120
    70+, 53, 74–77, 121
    day and night looks, 56–57, 60–61,
      64–65, 68–69, 72–73, 76–77
    overview, 52–53
Bags
    accenting LBD, 135
    choosing and buying, 198
    classics, 197
    enhancing eveningwear, 139, 143,
      152
    matching shoes with, 210–211
    for metallics and sequins, 143
    must-haves, 195
    for night brights, 139
    from office to cocktails, 152–153
    range of styles, 200–201
    for tuxedos, 147
    types of, 199
Basics, 9–27
    best investments, 16–17
    budget-saving finds, 18–19
    closet essentials, 10
    decision quandary and, 10
    optimizing wardrobe, 22–23
    timeless chic, 14–15

    ultimate classics, 12–13
    what to buy when, 24–25. *See also*
      Shopping
Belts, 123, 195, 212–213
Black dress. *See* Little black dress
  (LBD)
Blazers. *See* Jackets
Blouses. *See* Tops
Bohemian personalities, 35, 189
Bombshell personalities, 34
Boyish figures
    celebrating your shape, 86–87, 115,
      149
    perfect cocktail dress, 149
    perfect suit, 115
Bracelets, 218
Bras. *See* Lingerie
Brooches, 122, 219
Budget-saving finds, 18–19
Bust, balancing, 97
Calendar, shopping, 24–25
Career attire. *See* Office elegance
Casual chic, 155–191. *See also* Jeans;
  Tees, tanks, and turtlenecks;
  Weekend styles
    coats, 157, 178–181
    day dresses, 170–173
    jackets, 157, 166–169
    key pieces, 157
    knits, 157, 162–165
    layering pieces, 156, 158, 161
    overview, 156–157
    secrets of stylish women, 40–47
Classicist personalities, 33
Coats, 178–181
    best investment, 16
    casual chic, 157, 178–181
    how to wear, 180
    quantity needed, 20
    range of styles, 178–180
    trench, 99
    ultimate classic, 13
    universally flattering, 99
Cocktail attire. *See also* Evening glam
  and gowns
    from office to, 152–153
    perfect dress, 148–149
    secrets of stylish women, 40–47
Colorful eveningwear, 136–139
Country weekend style, 187

Curvy figures
    celebrating your shape, 82–83, 114,
      148
    perfect cocktail dress, 148
    perfect suit, 114
Day and night looks
    by age, 56–57, 60–61, 64–65,
      68–69, 72–73, 76–77
    by body shape, 83, 85, 87, 89, 91
Dressed-down dress-up, 150–151
Dresses. *See also* Evening glam and
  gowns; Little black dress (LBD)
    age-specific advice, 52–53, 54,
      58–59, 62–63, 66–67, 70–71
    balancing bust, 97
    basic essential, 11
    best investment, 17
    body shape and. *See* Shape,
      dressing for
    day, casual chic, 170–173
    for office, 112–113
    quantity needed, 20
    revealing/plunging necklines, 92–93
    showing shoulder, 96, 136–137
    timeless chic, 14
    ultimate classic, 12
    universally flattering, 98
    wrap, 99
Earrings, 216
Eclectic personalities, 39
Evening glam and gowns, 125–153.
  See also Little black dress (LBD)
    accessories accenting, 135, 139,
      143
    best investment, 17
    bright-colored dresses, 136–139
    dress codes and, 129
    dressed-down dress-up, 150–151
    from goddess to gamine, 130–131
    guidelines, 128–129
    overview, 126
    perfect cocktail dress, 148–149
    quick tips, 127
    range of styles, 130–131, 132–134,
      136–138, 140–142, 144–146,
      150–151
    revealing/plunging necklines, 92–93
    shape-specific advice, 148–149
    sparkling sequins and metallics,
      140–143

timeless allure, 130–131
tuxedos, 144–147
Extras. *See* Accessories
Fashion personalities, 32–39
  bohemians, 35
  bombshells, 34
  classicists, 33
  eclectics, 39
  ladies, 36
  mavericks, 37
  minimalists, 38
Figure, celebrating. *See* Shape,
  dressing for
Fuller figures
  celebrating your shape, 84–85, 115,
    149
  perfect cocktail dress, 149
  perfect suit, 115
Fur, 17
Glam weekend style, 184
Height, maximizing, 95
Jackets, 166–169
  age-specific advice, 52–53,
    55–56, 58, 62–63, 66–67, 70,
    74–75
  casual chic, 157, 166–169
  how to wear, 169
  quantity needed, 20
  range of styles, 166–168
  timeless chic, 14
  ultimate classic, 13
  ways to wear, 23
Jeans, 174–177
  basic essential, 11
  budget-saving finds, 18
  casual chic, 157, 174–177
  how to wear, 177
  quantity needed, 20
  range of styles, 174–176
  ultimate classics, 12
Jet-set weekend style, 188
Jewelry, 214–219
  accenting LBD, 135
  bracelets, 218
  brooches, 122, 219
  choosing, overview, 214
  classics, 196
  earrings, 122, 216
  enhancing eveningwear, 139, 143,
    147, 154

freshening up office basics, 122
for metallics and sequins, 143
must-haves, 195
necklaces, 122, 215
for night brights, 139
from office to cocktails, 152–153
rings, 217
for tuxedos, 147
Knits, 16, 162–165. *See also* Sweaters
  best investment, 16
  budget-saving finds, 19
  casual chic, 157, 162–165
  how to wear, 165
  optimizing use of, 22
  range of styles, 162–164
Lady personalities, 36
Lingerie, 221–231
  best basics, 226–227
  bra sizing, 223
  essential pieces, 224–225
  matching, 226
  proper fit, 222–223
  sexy staples, 228–229
  what to wear under what, 230–231
Little black dress (LBD), 132–135
  accessories accenting, 135
  as essential, 11
  range of styles, 132–134
  timeless chic, 14
  timelessness of, 132
Maverick personalities, 37
Metallics and sequins, 140–143
Minimalist personalities, 38
Necklaces, 122, 215
Office elegance, 101–123
  age-specific advice, 116–121
  basic essentials, 102
  dress code, 104–105
  dresses, 112–113
  freshening up basics, 122–123
  from office to cocktails, 152–153
  overview, 102–103
  pantsuits, 107, 108–109
  shape-specific advice, 114–115
  skirt suits, 107, 110–111
  suits, 106–111, 114–115
Pants and trousers. *See also* Jeans
  budget-saving finds, 18
  quantity needed, 20
  suits. *See* Suits

timeless chic, 14
ultimate classics, 12
Personal style, 29–49. *See also*
  Weekend styles
  age and. *See* Age-specific advice
  of Demi Moore, 46–47
  expert advice on finding, 48–49
  finding your own look, 31, 48–49
  goal for expressing, 30
  of Gwyneth Paltrow, 40–41
  of Nicole Kidman, 44–45
  personality categories. *See* Fashion
    personalities
  of professional designers, 48–49
  of Sarah Jessica Parker, 42–43
  secrets of stylish women, 40–47
  10 Commandments of Dressing,
    232–233
Petite figures
  celebrating your shape, 88–89, 115,
    149
  perfect cocktail dress, 149
  perfect suit, 115
Pregnancy
  celebrating your shape, 90–91, 115,
    149
  perfect cocktail dress, 149
  perfect suit, 115
Preppy weekend style, 183
Rings, 217
Rocker weekend style, 191
Romantic weekend style, 190
Sequins and metallics, 140–143
Shape, dressing for, 79–99
  accentuating your assets, 92–97
  age and. *See* Age-specific advice
  balancing bust, 97
  boyish figures, 86–87, 115, 149
  cocktail-dress selection, 148–149
  considerations, 81
  curvy figures, 82–83, 114, 148
  day and night looks, 83, 85, 87, 89,
    91
  defining waist, 94
  embracing your figure, 80
  fuller figures, 84–85, 115, 149
  maximizing height, 95
  petite figures, 88–89, 115, 149
  pregnancy and, 90–91, 115, 149
  revealing/plunging necklines, 92–93

showing shoulder, 96, 136–137
suit selection, 114–115
universally flattering pieces, 98–99
Shirts. *See* Tees, tanks, and
turtlenecks; Tops
Shoes
    accenting LBD, 135
    boot styles and selection, 206–209
    choosing and buying, 202, 206
    classics, 196, 197
    enhancing eveningwear, 139, 143,
      147, 153
    matching bags with, 210–211
    for metallics and sequins, 143
    must-haves, 195
    for night brights, 139
    from office to cocktails, 152–153
    range of styles, 204–205, 208–209
    for tuxedos, 147
    types of, 203, 207
Shopping, 26–27. *See also specific
items*
    budget-saving finds, 18–19
    calendar (what to buy when), 24–25
    time-saving tips, 27
Shoulder, showing, 96, 136–137
Skirts
    age-specific advice, 52–53,
      54–55, 58–59, 62–63, 66–67,
      70–71, 74–75
    basic essential, 11
    budget-saving finds, 18
    quantity needed, 20
    suits. *See* Suits
Sporty weekend style, 185
Suits
    age-specific advice, 116–121
    basic essential, 11
    black, 99
    freshening up basics, 122–123
    less conservative options, 116–121
    for office, 106–111
    optimizing use of, 22
    pantsuits, 107, 108–109, 114–115
    perfect, for your shape, 114–115
    quantity needed, 20
    skirt suits, 107, 110–111, 114–115
    timeless, tailored, 106
    universally flattering, 99
Sweaters. *See also* Knits
    quantity needed, 20
    ultimate classics, 12

Tees, tanks, and turtlenecks
    budget-saving finds, 19
    casual chic of, 157, 158–161
    how to wear, 161
    layering, 156, 158, 161
    optimizing use of, 22
    quantity needed, 20
    range of styles, 159–161
    ultimate classic, 12
10 Commandments of Dressing,
    232–233
Tops. *See also* Tees, tanks, and
turtlenecks
    age-specific advice, 52–53, 54–55,
      58–59, 62, 66, 70–71, 74–75
    basic essential, 11
    best investment, 17
    body shape and. *See* Shape,
      dressing for
    bright, freshening up basics, 123
    budget-saving finds, 19
    optimizing use of, 22
    quantity needed, 20
    white, 13
Trousers. *See* Pants and trousers
Tuxedo, 144–147
    accessories accenting, 147
    power and versatility, 144
    range of styles, 144–146
    timeless chic, 15
    ultimate classic, 13
Underwear. *See* Lingerie
Universally flattering pieces, 98–99
Urban weekend style, 186
Waist, defining/accentuating, 94
Wardrobe basics. *See* Basics
Weekend styles, 182–191
    bohemian, 189
    country, 187
    defining, 182
    glam, 184
    jet-set, 188
    preppy, 183
    rocker, 191
    romantic, 190
    sporty, 185
    urban, 186

Index of Personalities

Alba, Jessica, 167, 231
Aniston, Jennifer, 23, 33, 59, 141, 159
Armani, Giorgio, 17, 75, 101, 107, 211
Barkin, Ellen, 67
Barrymore, Drew, 14, 97, 151, 201, 218
Barton, Mischa, 54, 140, 158, 205
Beckham, Victoria, 217
Beene, Geoffrey, 221
Belle, Camilla, 169
Bello, Maria, 63, 160
Bening, Annette, 38
Berenson, Marisa, 71
Berry, Halle, 34, 82, 175, 197, 231
Biel, Jessica, 96, 231
Bilson, Rachel, 55, 132, 171, 201
Birkin, Jane, 35
Blahnik, Manolo, 193
Blair, Selma, 89, 133
Blanchett, Cate, 37, 103, 141
Blass, Bill, 155
Bosworth, Kate, 55
Bryant, Joy, 59, 117
Bullock, Sandra, 186
Burch, Tory, 113, 171, 212
Campbell, Naomi, 210
Carroll, Diahann, 75
Chanel, Coco, 9, 14, 196
Ciara, 176
Close, Glenn, 67
Collins, Joan, 98
Connelly, Jennifer, 37, 58, 183, 196
Coppola, Sofia, 59, 170, 196
Couric, Katie, 112
Crow, Sheryl, 63
Cruz, Penélope, 14, 106, 167
Danes, Claire, 149
Danner, Blythe, 71
Dawson, Rosario, 172
Dell'Orefice, Carmen, 75
Dench, Judi, 75
Deneuve, Catherine, 12, 71
Diaz, Cameron, 39, 99, 141, 157, 163,
    202
Dior, Christian, 51
Doillon, Lou, 122
Duff, Hilary, 174
Dunst, Kirsten, 35, 55, 131, 164
Ertegun, Mica, 75
Evangelista, Linda, 62
Ferrera, America, 85

Fonda, Jane; 70, 99
Foster, Jodie, 63
Fuentes, Daisy, 93
Gainsbourg, Charlotte, 123
Gyllenhaal, Maggie, 115
Haddon, Dayle, 67
Harlow, Shalom, 164
Harmon, Angie, 187
Hathaway, Anne, 116
Hepburn, Audrey, 14, 36, 196
Hepburn, Katharine, 14
Herrera, Carolina, 13, 48, 110, 120, 213
Holmes, Katie, 15, 91, 113, 179, 195
Hudson, Jennifer, 84, 149
Hudson, Kate, 35, 53, 123, 159, 208
Hurley, Elizabeth, 180
Huston, Anjelica, 99
Hutton, Lauren, 33, 71
Iman, 67, 119, 150
Jacobs, Marc, 59, 203
Jagger, Bianca, 15
Johansson, Scarlett, 94, 131, 163, 226
Jolie, Angelina, 38, 98
Karan, Donna, 49, 88, 93
Keaton, Diane, 39, 111
Kebede, Liya, 55
Kelly, Grace, 36, 197
Keys, Alicia, 93
Kidman, Nicole, 44–45, 213
Kikuchi, Rinko, 133
Klum, Heidi, 149
Knightley, Keira, 160, 189, 197
Knowles, Beyoncé, 133, 167
Kors, Michael, 55, 99, 108
Kruger, Diane, 113, 144, 180
Kurkova, Karolina, 188
Lagerfeld, Karl, 207
Lake, Veronica, 130
Lane, Diane, 92
Latifah, Queen, 114
Lauren, Ralph, 22
Laurent, Yves Saint, 29
Liu, Lucy, 89, 115, 178
Lohan, Lindsay, 55, 171, 209
Lopez, Jennifer, 34, 83, 130, 176, 184, 213
Loren, Sophia, 34, 92
Macpherson, Elle, 19, 33, 159, 223
Madonna, 37, 111, 137, 168, 185
Mainbocher, 79
Manheim, Camryn, 85
Marnay, Audrey, 173

McCartney, Stella, 108
McQueen, Alexander, 133
Mendes, Eva, 95
Miller, Sienna, 27, 35, 54, 94, 166, 215, 230
Minogue, Kylie, 206
Mirren, Helen, 71
Mizrahi, Isaac, 137
Monroe, Marilyn, 131
Moore, Demi, 14, 46–47, 196
Moore, Julianne, 63, 109
Moore, Mary Tyler, 75
Moss, Kate, 13, 31, 95, 145, 175, 197, 200
Murphy, Carolyn, 168, 180
Newton, Thandie, 59, 136
Olsen, Ashley, 55, 88, 151, 176, 219
Olsen, Mary-Kate, 162
Onassis, Jacqueline Kennedy, 14, 32, 197
Paltrow, Gwyneth, 11, 14, 40–41, 90, 111, 214
Parker, Sarah Jessica, 42–43, 95, 160, 205
Peet, Amanda, 177
Pickford, Mary, 131
Portman, Natalie, 86, 127
Posen, Zac, 141
Radziwill, Lee, 74, 121
Roberts, Julia, 145
Rodriguez, Narciso, 71
Russo, Rene, 67
Sawyer, Diane, 71, 96
Schiffer, Claudia, 161
Sedgwick, Kyra, 118
Sevigny, Chloë, 37, 59, 109, 151, 209
Simpson, Jessica, 34, 97, 175, 198, 231
Smith, Jada Pinkett, 149
Stefani, Gwen, 39, 58, 191
Stewart, Martha, 70
Stone, Sharon, 63
Streep, Meryl, 66
Swank, Hilary, 59, 97
Swinton, Tilda, 62
Taylor, Elizabeth, 34, 130, 196
Theron, Charlize, 38, 145, 228
Thomas, Kristin Scott, 63, 165
Thurman, Uma, 39, 179
Versace, Donatella, 49, 86, 199
Vreeland, Diana, 125
von Furstenberg, Diane, 48

Walters, Barbara, 75, 96
Wang, Vera, 67, 163
Washington, Kerry, 151, 172
Watts, Naomi, 109
Weaver, Sigourney, 66
Weisz, Rachel, 94, 172
Wek, Alek, 168
Williams, Michelle, 86, 137
Wilson, Rita, 164
Winfrey, Oprah, 83, 114, 180
Winslet, Kate, 38, 81, 99, 179
Witherspoon, Reese, 36, 91, 130, 137, 190, 213, 216
Wood, Natalie, 197
Wyatt, Lynn, 74
Zellweger, Renée, 36, 86, 115, 204
Zeta-Jones, Catherine, 110, 148

Photo Credits

CHAPTER 1

Page 8 Sølve Sundsbø; model: Carmen Kass. **Page 11** Scott Patterson/Big Pictures/Malibu Media. **Page 12** Courtesy Everett Collection. **Page 13** From left: Jennifer Graylock/FWD/Retna; Dennett/Knapik/Splash News. **Page 14** Clockwise from left: William Lovelace/Express/Getty Images; Marc Susset-Lacroix/WireImage; Lipnitzki/Roger Viollet/Getty Images; Grayson Alexander/Retna; courtesy Everett Collection; Splash News; Lalo Yasky/WireImage; Lester Glassner Collection/Neal Peters. **Page 15** From left: Peter Simins/*WWD*/Fairchild Publications, Inc.; Pierre Suu/Filmmagic. **Pages 16–19** Davies + Starr. **Page 23** From left: Luis Cavallari/Capital Pictures/Abaca USA; Arnaldo Magnani/Getty Images; Mario Anzuoni/Splash News. **Page 27** John Connor/Startraks Photo.

CHAPTER 2

Page 28 Terry Tsiolis; model: Caroline Trentini. **Page 31** Morrison-Huckle/Allaction/Retna. **Page 32** IPOL/Globe Photos. **Page 33** From left: INF Photo; Matrix/Bauer-Griffin; Michel Dufour. **Page 34** Clockwise from left: Fernando Allende/Splash News; Dimitrios Kambouris/WireImage; Globe Photos; Gregg DeGuire/WireImage; Frank Teti/Neal Peters Collection. **Page 35** From left: Gilbert Flores/Celebrity Photo; Omnia/Globe Photos; Jon Kopaloff/WireImage; INF Photo. **Page 36** From left: Lester Glassner Collection/Neal Peters; NPX/Starmax; John Kobal Foundation/Getty Images; Dimitrios Kambouris/WireImage. **Page 37** From left: Steve Granitz/WireImage; Rabbani and Solimene Photography/WireImage; Davidson/INF Photo; Sara De Boer/Retna. **Page 38** From left: Dimitrios Kambouris/WireImage; Vince Bucci/Getty Images; Eugene Gologursky/WireImage; Splash News. **Page 39** From left: Gregg DeGuire/WireImage; Peter Kramer/Getty Images; Steve Granitz/WireImage; Kevin Mazur/WireImage. **Page 40** INF Photo. **Page 41** From left: 626/Most Wanted/Zuma Press; Bauer-Griffin; Russ Einhorn/Splash News. **Page 42** Matt Baron/BEImages. **Page 43** From left: INF Photo; Arnaldo Magnani/Getty Images; Jamie McCarthy/WireImage. **Page 44** Scott Nelson/AFP/Getty Images. **Page 45** From left: INF Photo (2); Alberto Pizzoli/AFP/Getty Images. **Page 46** Jim Spellman/WireImage. **Page 47** From left: Gregg DeGuire/WireImage; Lisa Mauceri/INF Photo; Jeff Snyder/Filmmagic. **Page 48** From left: Duffy Marie Arnoult/WireImage; Jemal Countess/WireImage. **Page 49** From left: RJ Capak/WireImage; Rabbani and Solimene Photography/WireImage.

CHAPTER 3

Page 50 Alexi Lubomirski; model: Iselin Steiro. **Page 53** Euroimagen/LFI. **Page 54** From left: Jean-Paul Aussenard/WireImage; Ron Galella/WireImage. **Page 55** Clockwise from top left: Bennett Raglin/WireImage; Kevin Mazur/WireImage; Steve Granitz/WireImage; Patrick McMullan; Billy Farrell/Patrick McMullan; Stephen Shugerman/Getty Images. **Pages 56–57** Davies + Starr. **Page 58** From left: Bryan Bedder/Getty Images; Russ Einhorn/Splash News. **Page 59** Clockwise from top left: Theo Wargo/WireImage; Jim Rock/Abaca USA; Dimitrios Kambouris/WireImage; Gregg DeGuire/WireImage; Jemal Countess/WireImage; John Sciulli/WireImage. **Pages 60–61** Davies + Starr. **Page 62** From left: Rabbani & Solimene Photography/WireImage; Axelle/Bauer-Griffin. **Page 63** Clockwise from top left: Tony Barson/WireImage; Lester Cohen/WireImage; John Sciulli/WireImage; Patrick McMullan; Gregg DeGuire/WireImage; Jean Baptiste Lacroix/WireImage. **Pages 64–65** Davies + Starr. **Page 66** From left: Avik Gilboa/WireImage; David Lodge/WireImage. **Page 67** Clockwise from top left: Jamie McCarthy/WireImage; Steve Granitz/WireImage; Humberto Carreno/Startraks Photo; Amy Graves/WireImage; Steven Lovekin/WireImage; Jemal Countess/WireImage. **Pages 68–69** Davies + Starr. **Page 70** From left: Rabbani and Solimene Photography/WireImage; Frazer Harrison/Getty Images. **Page 71** Clockwise from top left: Kevin Mazur/WireImage; Patrick McMullan; Jaime Turner/Rex USA; RD/Leon/Retna; Michel Dufour/Getty Images; Donato Sardella/WireImage. **Page 72** Davies + Starr. **Page 73** Davies + Starr; Darryl Patterson. **Page 74** From left: Eric Ryan/Getty Images; Jamie McCarthy/WireImage. **Page 75** Clockwise from top left: Jamie McCarthy/WireImage; Dimitrios Kambouris/WireImage; Peter Kramer/Getty Images; Robert C. Mora/WireImage; Kevin Mazur/WireImage; John Barrett/Globe Photos. **Pages 76–77** Davies + Starr.

CHAPTER 4

Page 78 Karl Lagerfeld; models: Irina Lazareanu and Jessica Stam. **Page 81** Lisa O'Connor/Zuma Press. **Page 82** Steve Granitz/WireImage. **Page 83** From left: Mike Guastella/WireImage; Stephen Boitano/Getty Images. **Page 84** Sara De Boer/Retna. **Page 85** From left: John Sciulli/WireImage; Gregg DeGuire/WireImage. **Page 86** Frazer Harrison/Getty Images. **Page 87** From left: Koichi Kamoshida/Getty Images; Daniele Venturelli/WireImage. **Page 88** Steve Granitz/WireImage. **Page 89** From left: George Pimentel/WireImage; Scott Wintrow/Getty Images. **Page 90** Fotos International/Getty Images. **Page 91** From left: Clint Brewer/Splash News; Dave Benett/Getty Images. **Page 92** From left: George Pimentel/WireImage; Le Segretain/Getty Images. **Page 93** From left: Carlos Diaz/INF Photo; Dimitrios Kambouris/WireImage; Roger Wong/INF Photo. **Page 94** From left: Evan Agostini/Getty Images; Michael Germana/Starmax; Steve Granitz/WireImage. **Page 95** From left: Dara Kushner/INF Photo; Bauer-Griffin; Anna Polaro/Splash News. **Page 96** From left: Dimitrios Kambouris/WireImage; Peter Kramer/Getty Images; Eric Charbonneau/WireImage. **Page 97** From left: Jim Spellman/WireImage; George Pimentel/WireImage; Steve Granitz/WireImage. **Page 98** From left: Tomos Brangwyn/Retna; WireImage. Still life: Davies + Starr. **Page 99** From left: Steve Granitz/WireImage; Bauer-Griffin; Chris Polk/Filmmagic; Lawrence Lucier/Getty Images. Still life: Davies + Starr.

CHAPTER 5

Page 100 Tesh; model: Liya Kebede. **Page 103** Franziska Krug/Zuma Press. **Page 106** Eric Ryan/Getty Images. **Page 107** Eamonn McCormack/WireImage. Still life: Christopher Coppola. **Page 108** Russell Boyce/Landov. **Page 109** From left: INF Photo; Dimitrios Kambouris/WireImage (2). **Page 110** FTW/Starface/Retna. **Page 111** From left: INF Photo; Dimitrios Kambouris/WireImage; Claudio Guerrero/WireImage. **Page 112** Scott Wintrow/Getty Images. **Page 113** From left: Jaguar/AdMedia/Newscom; Erik T. Kaiser/Patrick McMullan; Rebecca Sapp/WireImage. **Page 114** Brad Barket/Getty Images. **Page 115** From left: Dara Kushner/INF Photo; Gregg DeGuire/WireImage; Djamilla Rosa Cochran/WireImage; Lester Cohen/WireImage. **Page 116** Billy Farrell/Patrick McMullan. Still life: Davies + Starr; Darryl Patterson. **Page 117** Noel Hines/Landov. Still life: Davies + Starr. **Page 118** Billy

Farrell/Patrick McMullan. Still life: Davies + Starr. **Page 119** Jamie McCarthy/WireImage. Still life: Davies + Starr; Darryl Patterson. **Page 120** Yuki Tanaka/LFI. Still life: Davies + Starr. **Page 121** Patrick McMullan. Still life: Davies + Starr; Darryl Patterson. **Page 122** Eric Ryan/Getty Images. Still life: Davies + Starr. **Page 123** From left: Andreas Rentz/Getty Images; FTW/Starface/Retna. Still life: Davies + Starr; Darryl Patterson.

CHAPTER 6
Page 124 Greg Kadel; model: Gisele Bündchen. **Page 127** George Pimentel/WireImage. **Page 130** From left: John Kobal Foundation/Getty Images; Lisa Rose/JPI Studios; courtesy Everett Collection; Jeff Vespa/WireImage. **Page 131** From left: Topical Press Agency/Getty Images; Peter Kramer/Getty Images; Photofest; Steve Granitz/WireImage. **Page 132** WireImage. **Page 133** From left: Barry King/WireImage; John Sciulli/WireImage; Kevin Mazur/WireImage. **Pages 134–135** Davies + Starr; Darryl Patterson. **Page 136** Gregg DeGuire/WireImage. **Page 137** From left: Frazer Harrison/Getty Images; George Pimentel/WireImage; Kevin Mazur/WireImage. **Pages 138–139** Davies + Starr. **Page 140** Jay Thornton/INF Photo. **Page 141** From left: Sean Gallup/Getty Images; James Devaney/WireImage; Lester Cohen/WireImage. **Pages 142–143** Davies + Starr; Darryl Patterson. **Page 144** Chris Jackson/Getty Images. **Page 145** From left: Chris Polk/Filmmagic; Nicolas Khayat/Abaca USA; Stephen Lovekin/WireImage. **Pages 146–147** Darryl Patterson; Davies + Starr. **Page 148** Dimitrios Kambouris/WireImage. **Page 149** From left: Dimitrios Kambouris/WireImage; Matthew Peyton/Getty Images; John Spellman/Retna; Donato Sardella/WireImage. **Page 150** Jamie

McCarthy/WireImage. **Page 151** From left: John Sciulli/WireImage; Jamie McCarthy/WireImage; George Pimentel/WireImage; Jim Spellman/WireImage. **Pages 152-153** Davies + Starr.

CHAPTER 7
Page 154 Greg Kadel; model: Gemma Ward. **Page 157** Jun Sato/WireImage. **Page 158** BBH/INF Photo. **Page 159** From left: James Devaney/WireImage; Splash News; INF Photo. **Page 160** From left: Dara Kushner/INF Photo; Donato Sardella/WireImage; Jon Beretta/Rex USA. **Page 161** Anthony Harvey/WireImage. **Page 162** Splash News. **Page 163** From left: Scott Gries/Getty Images; Jason Kempin/Filmmagic; Uno Press/WireImage. **Page 164** From left: Jean-Paul Aussenard/WireImage; Jeff Steinberg/INF Photo; Theo Wargo/WireImage. **Page 165** Mike Marsland/WireImage. **Page 166** Steve Granitz/WireImage. **Page 167** From left: Steve Granitz/WireImage; Semmer/Face to Face/Abaca USA; Mario Magnani/Getty Images. **Page 168** From left: Jean-Paul Aussenard/WireImage; Humberto Carreno/Startraks Photo; Jean Baptiste Lacroix/WireImage. **Page 169** Chris Weeks/WireImage. **Page 170** Fitzroy Barrett/Globe Photos. **Page 171** From left: Daniele Venturelli/WireImage; Lionel Hahn/Abaca USA; James Devaney/WireImage. **Page 172** From left: Stephen Lovekin/WireImage; Tony Barson/WireImage; Peter Kramer/Getty Images. **Page 173** David Lodge/WireImage. **Page 174** Jean Baptiste Lacroix/WireImage. **Page 175** From left: Jeff Steinberg/INF Photo; Gregg DeGuire/WireImage; Dave M. Bennett/Getty Images. **Page 176** From left: Brad Barket/Getty Images; Jemal Countess/WireImage; Vickers/Whittle/Splash News. **Page 177** Steve Granitz/WireImage. **Page 178** Lee Roth/Starmax. **Page 179** From left: Roger Wong/INF/Starmax;

Bryan Bedder/Getty Images; Pegasus/Splash News. **Page 180** Eric Ryan/Getty Images; Ronald Asadorian/Splash News; Dimitrios Kambouris/WireImage. **Page 181** Arnaldo Magnani/Getty Images. **Page 183** Roger Wong/INF Photo. Still life: Darryl Patterson; Davies + Starr; Roger Cabello. **Page 184** Bill Davila/Startraks Photo. Still life: Davies + Starr; Darryl Patterson. **Page 185** Ian Lawrence/Splash News. Still life: Darryl Patterson; Davies + Starr. **Page 186** Humberto Carreno/Startraks Photo. Still life: Davies + Starr. **Page 187** Peter Kramer/Getty Images. Still life: Darryl Patterson; Davies + Starr. **Page 188** Kyriazis Stefanos/Startraks Photo. Still life: Davies + Starr; Darryl Patterson; Christopher Coppola. **Page 189** Bauer-Griffin. Still life: Davies + Starr; Darryl Patterson; Christopher Coppola. **Page 190** Steve Granitz/WireImage. Still life: Darryl Patterson; Davies + Starr. **Page 191** John Beretta/Rex USA. Still life: Davies + Starr; Darryl Patterson.

CHAPTER 8
Page 192 Anthony Ward; model: Valentina Zelyaeva. **Page 195** Bauer-Griffin. **Page 196** Clockwise from left: Paramount/Neal Peters Collection; Bryan Bedder/Getty Images; courtesy Everett Collection; Jim Spellman/WireImage; Michael Caulfield/WireImage; Lipnitzki/Roger Viollet/Getty Images. **Page 197** Clockwise from left: Retro/Villard/Sipa Press; Ian Millar/Splash News; *Evening Standard*/Getty Images; Bauer-Griffin/M. Barazza/Wenn/Newscom; courtesy Everett Collection. **Page 198** Dara Kushner/INF Photo. **Page 199** Davies + Starr; Christopher Coppola. **Page 200** Bauer-Griffin. Still life: Davies + Starr. **Page 201** From left: Bauer-Griffin; Humberto Carreno/Startraks Photo. Still life: Davies + Starr. **Page 202** Steve Granitz/WireImage. **Page 203**

Darryl Patterson; Davies + Starr. **Page 204** Starmax. Still life: Darryl Patterson. **Page 205** From left: Nick Harvey/WireImage; Dimitrios Kambouris/WireImage. Still life: Davies + Starr. **Page 206** Goff/Whitaker/INF Photo. **Page 207** Darryl Patterson; Davies + Starr. **Page 208** Splash News. Still life: Davies + Starr. **Page 209** From left: Thornton/Mauceri/INF Photo; London Entertainment/Splash News. Still life: Davies + Starr. **Page 210** Michael Swarbrick/INF Photo. **Page 211** Davies + Starr; Darryl Patterson. **Page 212** Rabbani and Solimene Photography/WireImage. **Page 213** From left: James Devaney/WireImage; Kevin Mazur/WireImage; Stefanie Keenan/Patrick McMullan. Still life: Darryl Patterson; Davies + Starr. **Page 214** George Pimentel/WireImage. Still life: Davies + Starr. **Page 215** Dave Hogan/Getty Images. Still life: Davies + Starr. **Page 216** Kevin Winter/Getty Images. Still life: Christopher Coppola; Darryl Patterson; Davies + Starr. **Page 217** Evan Agostini/Getty Images. Still life: Davies + Starr; Darryl Patterson. **Page 218** Gregg DeGuire/WireImage. Still life: Darryl Patterson; Davies + Starr. **Page 219** Goff/INF. Still life: Davies + Starr; Darryl Patterson.

CHAPTER 9
Page 220 Terry Tsiolis; model: Hilary Rhoda. **Page 223** Splash News. **Page 226** Jeffrey Mayer/WireImage. **Page 227** Davies + Starr; Christopher Coppola; Darryl Patterson. **Page 228** Alistair Linford/Rex USA. **Page 229** Darryl Patterson; Davies + Starr. **Page 230** Jon Furniss/WireImage. Still life: Davies + Starr. **Page 231** From left: Andrew Rocke/INF Photo; Eric Charbonneau/WireImage; James Devaney/WireImage; Dimitrios Kambouris/WireImage. Still life: Darryl Patterson; Davies + Starr; Chris Bartlett.

Library of Congress Cataloging-in-Publication Data
Levin, Jenny.
 Harper's bazaar great style: best ways to update your look / Jenny Levin.
    p. cm.
 Includes index.
 ISBN-13: 978-1-58816-673-9
 ISBN-10: 1-58816-673-2
 1. Fashion. 2. Beauty, Personal. 3. Women's clothing. 4. Lifestyles. I. Harper's bazaar II. Title. III. Title: Great style.
 TT507.L448 2007
 746.9'2--dc22

                         2007007867

10 9 8 7 6 5 4 3 2

Designers: Elsa Mehary, Gary Ponzo
Photo Editor: Leyla Sharabi
Digital Imaging Specialists: Peter Rundqvist, Aaron Bitters
Managing Editor: Nancy Gillen
Copy Editor: Sarah Strzelec
Production: Tom McKee
Consulting Editors: Sarah Bailey, Kristina O'Neill

Published by Hearst Books
A Division of Sterling Publishing Co., Inc.
387 Park Avenue South, New York, NY 10016

Harper's Bazaar and Hearst Books are trademarks of Hearst Communications, Inc.

www.harpersbazaar.com

For information about custom editions, special sales, premium, and corporate purchases,
please contact Sterling Special Sales Department at 800-805-5489 or specialsales@sterlingpub.com.

Distributed in Canada by Sterling Publishing
c/o Canadian Manda Group, 165 Dufferin Street
Toronto, Ontario, Canada M6K 3H6

Manufactured in China

Sterling ISBN 13: 978-1-58816-673-9
        ISBN 10: 1-58816-673-2